BOUNTIFUL,
BEAUTIFUL,
BLISSFUL

BOUNTIFUL, BEAUTIFUL, BLISSFUL

Experience the Natural Power of Pregnancy and Birth with Kundalini Yoga

GURMUKH

FOREWORD BY *Cindy Crawford*

MICHAEL JOSEPH
an imprint of
PENGUIN BOOKS

MICHAEL JOSEPH

Published by the Penguin Group
Penguin Books Ltd, 80 Strand, London WC2R 0RL, England
Penguin Putnam Inc., 375 Hudson Street, New York, New York 10014, USA
Penguin Books Australia Ltd, 250 Camberwell Road, Camberwell, Victoria 3124, Australia
Penguin Books Canada Ltd, 10 Alcorn Avenue, Toronto, Ontario, Canada M4V 3B2
Penguin Books India (P) Ltd, 11 Community Centre, Panchsheel Park, New Delhi - 110 017, India
Penguin Books (NZ) Ltd, Cnr Rosedale and Airborne Roads, Albany, Auckland, New Zealand
Penguin Books (South Africa) (Pty) Ltd, 24 Sturdee Avenue, Rosebank 2196, South Africa

Penguin Books Ltd, Registered Offices: 80 Strand, London WC2R 0RL, England

www.penguin.com

First published in the United States of America by St Martin's Press 2003
First published in Great Britain by Michael Joseph 2003
1

Grateful acknowledgement is made to Yogi Bhajan for permission to reprint his poem
'The Law of Love' on page v.
Photo on page v courtesy of Dawn Baillie/BLT & Associates, Inc.

Printed in Great Britain by Clays Ltd, St Ives plc

A CIP catalogue record for this book is available from the British Library

THE LAW OF LOVE

LOVE GIVES YOU POWER TO MERGE,

FROM FINITE TO INFINITY.

LOVE GIVES YOU POWER TO TRUST,

FROM NOTHING TO EVERYTHING.

LOVE GIVES YOU POWER, THE POWERFUL PRAYER

BETWEEN YOU AND YOUR CREATOR.

LOVE GIVES YOU VASTNESS,

AS VAST AS THERE CAN BE.

LOVE GIVES YOU THE HOLD, THE EXPERIENCE,

AND THE TOUCH WITH YOUR OWN INFINITY,

AS BEAUTIFUL, BOUNTIFUL AND BLISSFUL AS THERE CAN BE.

—— YOGI BHAJAN

CONTENTS

FOREWORD

I came to Gurmukh through a friend of mine who had been a student of hers for years and swore by her teaching. When I became pregnant with my first child, my friend told me, "You *have* to take this class. It will be great for you and the baby." She was so enthusiastic that she actually went to my first prenatal yoga class with me, and she wasn't even pregnant!

It's impossible to tell you everything I took away from the experience of going to Gurmukh's prenatal classes, because there was just so much. One of the first things that struck me was the sense of community among the pregnant women. There is nothing like sharing time with women who are in the exact same place you are. No matter who you are, having your baby is the most important thing in the world at that point in your life, and that unites you with every other pregnant woman. It was such an incredible time for me, and everyone in my class became really good friends. We're still close. In fact, we jokingly call ourselves the "yoga babies group" and continue to get together every week, even though we've all long since given birth (and half of us are on number two).

The ideas and issues about pregnancy and childbirth raised by Gurmukh and the other women in class were wonderful catalysts for conversation. I found that it was a great place to share information and for questions to be raised. The topics we discussed in class spurred me to do my own research and investigate other options besides the conventional childbirth experience.

What I learned put me on the path to having a home birth, which was the most transforming experience of my life. When I became pregnant, I assumed I would simply go to the hospital, sign up for an epidural, and that would be that. I thought that's just how everyone did it. I didn't even know women had babies at home anymore. Through referrals in my yoga class, I found incredible midwives who were there to help and guide me, but what I found so meaningful about working with them was that they never tried to "manage" me or contain my labor within some predetermined experience. I recently had my second child, again at home. Though this birth was so different from the birth of my son, what the two experiences had in common was that the midwives did not try to control the process or make it into something other than what it was. They allow your birth to be *your* birth.

A big part of why I did decide on a home birth was the faith and trust I got from Gurmukh that women's bodies contain the knowledge and the fortitude to bring children into the world. Knowing that I am part of a long lineage of women who have experienced the same dramatic event not only kept me from being terrified of the process, but gave me the confidence in myself as a woman and in my body's natural ability, as well as the tools I needed, to deal with natural childbirth.

My advice to you? First, go hang out with other pregnant women. If you don't have a yoga class or another group in your area, get one of Gurmukh's videos, find other pregnant women, and invite them over! It's so important to be around others who are going through the same changes and feelings as you. Only another pregnant woman will let you talk about it for as long as you need to talk about it.

Second, and perhaps most important, don't wish your pregnancy away. Whatever you're going through, you will never be in that particular moment again. During the first few weeks of pregnancy, don't wish you could already feel the baby move. If you can already feel the baby move, don't wish you were already giving birth. Don't wish to be any place other than where you are. Even when you're feeling morning sick, enjoy that time. Enjoy the time during the last few weeks before your due date when you feel nervous and jittery with anticipation. Enjoy it all, because every moment is part of the experience.

Honestly, I wasn't one of those women who loved being pregnant, in the sense that I didn't feel I was at my sexiest or most beautiful, as some do. In Gurmukh's class, there would always be a point at which we would sit with our hands around our bellies and sing to our babies. In that moment, I always felt the tremendous power we as women have to bring new life into the world. It's awe-inspiring.

Finally, I want to say a few things about Gurmukh herself. It's unfortunate the whole world can't come to her class and feel her energy directly—although sometimes it feels like it, her classes are that popular! Her radiance lights up a room. The strength and confidence she imparts to us is just so wonderful. I have no doubt the essence of her wisdom and caring will be filtered to you as you read these pages.

I wish you all the best for your journey into motherhood.

— CINDY CRAWFORD

A PROGRAM
FOR LIFE

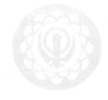

When a child comes into your life, it is as if a small stone is thrown into a pool. You will see the ripples spread outward, touching not only your own existence but that of your immediate family, your friends and extended family, your community, and, ultimately, the entire planet.

The Khalsa Way, the name of the program we teach at Golden Bridge, our center in Los Angeles, is based in this simple metaphor. The program is rooted in the ancient science and techniques of Kundalini yoga and meditation, a yogic practice developed to provide the most profound results in the shortest possible time to families and individuals. More than a prenatal yoga class, The Khalsa Way is a program for life that addresses childbirth education and parenting, as well as community-awareness issues.

Birth is possibly the greatest time of transformation in your life: A baby is born, a woman is born as a mother, a man as a father, a family as a family. From this point forward the ripples reach out to touch the community at large.

What you'll find in these pages is a blueprint for emotional, physical, and spiritual health for the nine months of pregnancy and beyond. I offer it to you regardless of whether you are simply thinking about having a child, actively trying to conceive, or are pregnant with your first baby or your fifth. The book is broken into sections that cover the trimesters of pregnancy, delivery, and life with baby. In each section you'll find little chapters offering inspiration, advice, and information to help you along the way.

At every point in the journey of motherhood, you'll face many opportunities to grow and strengthen yourself, your baby, your relationship, your family, your contributions to your community, and, above all, your spirit. This book offers you tools to help you explore and, when necessary, heal your own history and unconscious attitudes about pregnancy, birth, and parenting. These tools will help you develop an even deeper, more conscious bond with the soul growing inside you. And like that ripple from a pond, this swells to include more fully your partner and other children in the process, and honor the connection among all of you.

My intention is also to provide you with information to which you have not had access: knowledge about birthing and infant care that isn't in the mainstream of today's Western culture, but which has been around literally for eons. With knowledge comes true choice, and my wish is that you and your family have all you need to choose consciously what will best suit your physical, emotional, and spiritual needs.

I encourage you to use this book in the way that makes sense for you. Read this book in the traditional manner from beginning to end, or skip around among the sections to read chapters that match what you feel are your physical and emotional needs at the moment. Above all, listen to yourself. Perhaps you will choose several of the many exercises and meditations and concentrate on those, or decide to do one of them as a forty-day commitment. Another way is simply to hold the book in your hands, shut your eyes, and say a little prayer, calling upon God in whatever form you understand God to be, to work through your intuition to give you the guidance you need at the moment. Then, allow the book to open wherever it will and read the page it lands on. Be willing to consider that wherever the book has opened is the message you need right now. Let that be your focus for the day. This is how I always approach books I find inspiring, and I never fail to find exactly the answer I am seeking.

BLESSINGS,

GURMUKH

YOGA AND MEDITATION DIRECTORY

INTRODUCTION

"White-Shell-Woman, she moves . . .
Before her all is beautiful,
she moves,
Behind her all is beautiful,
she moves."

—NAVAJO SONG

I have been a yoga and meditation teacher for thirty-two years, and I continually witness the incredible power of this ancient science to uplift the spirit and heal mind and body. Yoga literally means "to yoke," that is, to join yourself to the Infinite. The essence of yoga is about relationship, and nowhere is this more true than during pregnancy, when your life is in every sense joined to your baby's. Each week at Golden Bridge, our yoga center in Los Angeles, hundreds of women and families attend the prenatal and postnatal yoga classes and childbirth education courses. The mothers and fathers come because they're committed to having a healthy pregnancy, but what always makes me smile is to watch their growing realization that preparing for the birth of a child is really about preparing for the rest of life as a parent. Yoga is a state of receptivity from which we can begin to learn and make lasting changes.

Having a child is a beautiful kind of alchemy. What this soul brings to you, and what you bring to the soul, transforms you both for all time. I'm not exaggerating when I tell you teaching pregnant women is my greatest passion in life. Having a child is a living prayer and simply amazing grace. Our power as women to form another life within our bodies is almost too vast to comprehend. In our current culture, we too often forget this is a sacred miracle. I learned this important lesson long ago from a young girl named Mary.

As a child, Mary was quiet and had quite an imagination. She could spend many hours sitting by a window, daydreaming as she gazed outside, or playing with her dollies. Because of her reserved nature, her family dubbed her "Mary Sit-and-Do-Nothing," a nickname that made her feel she was a disappointment to them. She also assumed that she must not be very smart and that something must be wrong with her because she was the only person she knew who liked to be quiet. She grew up in the forties and fifties when action equaled success. No one had even heard the word "meditate" in her small Illinois farm town.

In the early 1960s, when she was in her teens, Mary's sister had been prescribed diet pills by a doctor as a way to lose weight, a common practice in those days. The doctor didn't say the medicine was an addictive amphetamine. When Mary's sister suggested that she take them, too, because they provided "energy," she happily agreed and soon had her own prescription. The pills made her mind race, her weight drop, and did indeed fill her with a frenetic energy. "Wow! Now I'm Mary-Do-Everything!" she thought to herself. She could now fulfill her parents' dream of her as a productive girl just like the rest.

Mary soon became addicted to this drug. Even though the word "addiction" was not used in American culture at the time, she knew she couldn't get through a day without them. She kept that realization a secret. After all, to whom could she really talk about this? No one she knew.

At age nineteen, Mary left her small town in Illinois to attend college at San Francisco State University in California. She couldn't get her out-of-state prescription filled in California. At first she panicked, but then it hit her that she must stop. So she did. For almost a year she felt sick and listless from her abrupt withdrawal from the drug. When she slept, her mind was plagued with nightmares.

Eventually, she met a man and fell in love. He was older than she by a dozen years and a Ph.D. student. She saw in him a wiser, dependable man whom she wanted to believe would fill her father's place; he'd died a slow and painful death from cancer several months before Mary fell in love with this man.

When she realized she was pregnant, Mary didn't know what to do. She was twenty-one years old. Calling her conservative family to explain she'd gotten pregnant was a stressful, shame-filled experience because she felt she'd let them down. Although neither of them felt ready for marriage, she and her boyfriend both believed they had no other option. Abortion was not legal, and there was no place in society for an unwed mother. It was a painful, confusing time, but she also was elated at the prospect of a new life growing inside her.

She looked for an OB/GYN in the San Francisco Yellow Pages, deciding on the one who was closest to where she lived. She wanted to like him, she wanted to trust him, but she did not. He was the kind of doctor who didn't even say hello when he walked into his office, and he'd make insensitive comments like, "If you put on any more weight we won't be able to wheel you into the delivery room, because you won't fit through the door." She felt humiliated. Without her diet pills, she no longer felt that false sense of self-esteem drugs provide, let alone the energy or the "I can do anything" feeling. She was on a downward spiral of feeling fat and ugly, and the doctor seemed to confirm the bad feelings she had about herself.

Mary cried and cried after her visits to his office, explaining to her husband how afraid she was of this doctor. Still, it didn't occur to either one of them that they had a choice to change doctors. It was as if he were a god they dared not defy. So with a stiff upper lip she marched herself back each week to the doctor's office, feeling like a failure on all counts.

She went into labor on November 4, 1964, during the election in which Jerry Brown was running for governor of California. Her husband wasn't allowed to come with her when they wheeled her into the delivery room, where a television blared, because the staff did not want to miss the gubernatorial election returns. She was put flat on her back on a delivery table with her feet up in stirrups. Without saying anything or asking permission, the anesthesiologist gave her a shot in the back with a very long needle. Years later, she would understand that she had been given an epidural without her consent.

As she labored, the anesthesiologist was the only person who asked her questions. He held her hand. She thought he alone cared about her. Not until years later did she realize the only reason he was talking to her was to gauge how the anesthesia was working. She would always remember his hand over hers, because it was the only thing real in an otherwise uncaring room. The walls were a cold green, and she barely saw the faces above her because they were all watching the TV screen over their shoulders to see what the latest returns were. Their conversation was, of course, about who was going to win. Meanwhile Mary lay below the politics and the small talk, praying to have some help, some comfort, some reassurance that everything was going to be all right, and that she could do it. None came.

And that is how her baby came into the world.

Mary was too naïve, ignorant, and scared to demand that her needs be met. In fact, she didn't even know *what* her needs were—that's how far removed she was from her own feelings. She'd never heard about yoga, childbirth education classes, or books about pregnancy. Finally, she slipped into unconsciousness, and had no memory of how the child, a baby boy, was pulled from her.

After three days in the hospital—considered a usual stay back then—Mary prepared to go home with her son, a seven-pound, four-ounce boy named Shannon Danuele. She had started nursing him, despite the fact that no one encouraged her to do it. The hospital staff supplied her with bottles and formula, but she knew in her heart that nursing was what she needed to do, because her mother had nursed her.

One thing she knew for certain: She didn't want circumcision for her son. She didn't even know what an uncircumcised boy would look like—the men in her family, her husband, even the children she baby-sat as a teenager, were all circumcised. Yet she couldn't see the reason her son should have to go through the pain of having a natural part of his body cut off. She told the doctor that she thought the practice was unnecessary and a little barbaric. He hit the roof.

"You'll create a monster who will hate you for not having this done!" he told her. "I refuse to release this child until you come to your senses."

She cried, she begged, but she felt she could not fight. Once again the god had spoken, and she was wrong. She finally agreed so she could take her baby and go home.

Eleven days after he was born, Shannon went into cardiac arrest. He had been born with a congenital heart defect. Mary and her husband struggled to keep their boy alive. Shannon could not cry, because his heart would stop. Many nights the couple would take their Volkswagen van and drive the empty streets of San Francisco, going up and down the steep hills to keep Shannon from crying. Although he had a hard time sucking, Mary continued to nurse him, supplementing with formula from a bottle. She hardly put him down, so she herself slept and ate little, but she was on a mission. The doctors said if Shannon could be kept alive until age two, they could perform a surgery that would save his life.

He did not make it to age two. At seven months, Shannon left his body and went back to the timeless place souls go. He died in the hospital while Mary had gone home to get a couple hours' sleep. No chance to hold him in her arms for the last time. She didn't even get to say good-bye.

The day after he died, Mary's husband was scheduled to go north to where he was doing his internship for a Ph.D. in clinical psychology. He asked her if he should go. "Don't worry," she assured him, "I'll be fine." And so she was left alone. She had no words for the pain she felt, no way to express her insanity, rage, and sadness. All that she knew was a mute, aching void inside her. She was vaguely aware of her hands tearing at her scalp, pulling her hair straight up to the sky, screaming, "No! No!" What had she done? Was there no one who could talk to her and help her? For days she ceaselessly walked a circular pattern around the silent, empty apartment, but even the constant movement could bring no relief from her agony, loss, and guilt.

She had no tools to help her grieve, no way to transcend her isolation. It took Mary many years to understand fully how relinquishing all of her power to others and ignoring her own gut instincts had led to such a tragic outcome.

I know this feeling all too well. You see, Mary "Sit-and-Do-Nothing" was me.

 In my own experience, and in the experience of many other women who have shared their stories with me over the years, I find that along with the life-saving advances available in our modern high-tech medical system come some difficult challenges for the pregnant and laboring woman. Women's knowledge about themselves, their bodies, and their feelings is not only overlooked, but can be discredited outright in the authoritarian tradition of Western medicine. Sometimes the only information taken seriously is what comes from doctors and controlled clinical studies. Women often assume if they want to be a modern, responsible mother, they need to discount what they are feeling and the conclusions they arrive at intuitively. The mission of my life is to see no more women and children suffer the kind of ignorance and pain that I knew with my first baby.

I have come to know that God makes no mistakes. Every life has a profound purpose. I believe that my baby boy was brought as a kind of guardian angel, because without him I would not have been led to seek healing, and I might have missed my own destiny, which is to share with you the profound wisdom and science of Kundalini Yoga and Meditation as taught by Yogi Bhajan. With this wisdom of the ancient ones, you can begin to experience your own truest nature. If you know how to be human, you know how to be a mother—how to be anything and everything!

Eventually, my first husband and I divorced. It was not a mean parting, just a sad one. For years afterwards, I was still longing to belong; the sadness in me from the death of my first child and a lifelong feeling of not fitting in or knowing my purpose made me question why I was here on this earth, and what it was all about. I traveled the world, as if by logging thousands of miles I could somehow find what I was longing for—me. When I think back on it now, I was really on a spiritual quest, looking for answers to life's greatest questions. I was searching to find my people, my tribe, my home.

From living in Haight Ashbury, I went to Big Sur, then took off to hitchhike my way through Mexico and lived among the native people there. After that, I lived on a beach in Maui for two years as a hippie, dancing, chanting, fasting, doing hallucinogenic drugs, body surfing, and owning nothing. A noncommitted life was what I defined as freedom in comparison to the strictness of my upbringing. Eventually

God led me to a Zen Buddhist zendo where I sat zazen, a rigorous form of silent meditation, for seven hours a day with no drugs, and celibate, for a year. In fact, I thought I would become a Zen nun and was on my way back to the mainland for a visit home before starting my training in Japan. I had no idea what was actually in store for me.

By then it was 1970. Once again, through the amazing grace of God, I was led to an ashram in Arizona that practiced Kundalini yoga and meditation. I had run into an old friend while I was in Big Sur—actually, he sought me out on his twenty-first birthday, because he said he had a vivid dream in which God told him he was supposed to take me to an ashram in Arizona. Ashram? I didn't even know what the word meant. He was someone I trusted, and he was adamant that God had given him direct orders too powerful to ignore, so I thought, well, why not? I had been living in the flow of things for years at that point. I could easily delay my trip to Japan for a few days. We packed up his little Volkswagen bug and headed to Tucson, not knowing what lay ahead.

Once we arrived, he paid seventy-five dollars for a month's room and board for me at the ashram. He stayed and meditated for seven days, and then simply drove off to I don't know where. I never saw him again. I don't know how I can explain this, but the minute I walked through the doors of the ashram, I felt a peaceful feeling flow through me, as if I had done all this before. That day I found my true dharma, or life path. The weary traveler had finally come home. That was more than three decades ago.

My spiritual teacher, Yogi Bhajan, brought the technology of Kundalini yoga and meditation to the West. For thousands of years, this was a mystical practice passed in secret from master to student, but Yogi Bhajan lifted the veil of secrecy and made this powerful technology available to everyday people living in communities where once only ascetics knew it. The lives of families and whole communities have benefited by being uplifted and made joyful, healthful, and fulfilled. It was he who gave me my spiritual name, Gurmukh, which means "one who helps thousands cross the world oceans." He also told me that I would help deliver babies.

At first I took this quite literally. While living at an ashram in northern New Mexico, I apprenticed myself to an OB/GYN doctor in Santa Fe who did home births, volunteering to clean his house and office in exchange for attending births and learning from him all that I could about birthing. It was an amazing, divine experience to see souls take their first breath in the world, and I learned so much about life helping to bring in these souls and about our power as women—so different from what I had experienced giving birth to Shannon. I couldn't see myself becoming a midwife, and so eventually my studies trailed off as teaching yoga became more of my full-time occupation.

In 1977 I went to India on a *yatra*, or spiritual pilgrimage, and upon my return I moved to Los Angeles, where I finally met my soul mate and spiritual partner, Gurushabd Singh. We married in the fall of 1982. We would rise every morning at 3:30 A.M. to begin *sadhana*, our daily practice of prayer, yoga, and meditation. I had visions that I would conceive, and it would be on May 15. I still remember it so vividly that when I shut my eyes it's like a movie playing in my head. I was in my early forties, and thought that becoming pregnant would be difficult. But, sure enough, on May 15, 1983, when I was forty-two, we conceived our daughter, twenty years after my son was born. It was God's miracle made manifest.

At the time, I could find only one exercise class for pregnant women in Los Angeles. I went, but it wasn't very nurturing or cheery. I felt fat and awkward and out of place. We didn't talk or get cozy; we just listened to really brash music and moved as if we were in an exercise aerobics class. Then I found a regular stretch class with an instructor named Peter at the Jane Fonda Studio, a wonderful exercise facility within walking distance from my home. Peter was so kind and supportive, and became dear to me all through my pregnancy. As my belly got larger, he geared the class to me. At the end, when the class did abdominal work, I would give Peter a hug of thanks and then stroll home, knowing that abs were not for me. I was so happy I went almost every day, so much did I love being in a class with others.

Being a yoga teacher, I devised a program of my own. I walked every day, used Kundalini yoga sets Yogi Bhajan recommended for pregnancy, and continued with my meditation. I think God's grace and this program were to thank for the fact that my giving birth at forty-three years of age was challenging, but certainly not impossible.

In February 1984, I gave birth to our daughter, Wahe Guru Kaur, in our family bed at home with the help of a midwife. Unlike the experience of naïve young Mary, this experience of labor was of one long meditation, a continual spiral inward that opened my body as the petals of a flower open under the warmth of the sun. At least, that's my memory of it. A couple years ago, someone asked me if I cried out during labor, and I confidently shook my head no. My husband looked at me as if I was crazy and said, "What are you talking about? You yelled your lungs out!" Oh, well. I truly had no memory of that, because I was on a deep inner journey, beyond words.

Students and strangers alike wanted to know what I did during my pregnancy. It dawned on me that I did know a few things I could offer, so I began to teach a small group of pregnant women yoga classes in my tiny home—we called it the "bird's nest" because it was cute and snug—with baby Wa asleep in the next room. Soon there were more and more women lining up at my door, hungry to be taught a different approach to pregnancy than what was typically available. We had to find a bigger house to accommodate the demand for classes!

Today, nineteen years later, hundreds of women attend yoga and The Khalsa Way, our childbirth education program, and couples' classes held each week at Golden Bridge. Most mamas return forty days after their babies are born for the Mommy and Me classes. Dads are so very welcomed. It's become an ever-extending family. After all these years, I have come to appreciate exactly what Yogi Bhajan meant when he decreed I would deliver babies: He meant that I would help deliver souls into the arms of mothers who are physically, mentally, and spiritually prepared to guide them on their amazing trip through this lifetime.

Yogi Bhajan came to America not to gather students but to create teachers. In that spirit, our Khalsa Way Teachers Training attracts women from all over the world who come to study one week for sixty hours to earn training certification. These women take the teachings to their communities and spread the word. This means these ancient teachings are helping women and families throughout the world, and ultimately the world itself.

Our job as parents is to raise our consciousness not only about conception, pregnancy, delivery, and parenting, but also about our own lives. Our duty is to give children what they need in life so that they will always remember who they are: *spiritual beings born to have a human experience.*

Our bodies are the means by which we come to know and cherish our connection to the Infinite. Our practice is to awaken the Kundalini, the primal energy that rests at the base of our spine, like the coils of a sleeping snake. Kundalini yoga, like the sound of the Indian flute player raising the cobra from its slumber, moves this energy up our spine by means of *asanas* (postures), *pranayama* (breath control), *mudra* (hand positions that stimulate centers in your brain), and *mantra* (repetitive sounds we make to bring about a change in our consciousness).

When this yoga is practiced, even in a simple form, we are not only strengthening our physical body but are also stimulating and balancing our chakra system. Chakra is the Sanskirt word for "wheel." Think of your chakras as spinning vortexes of energy throughout your body, each radiating a particular energy that is important for your health, happiness, and well-being. How does this actually work? Think of the energy of your body's extensive glandular system combining with your central nervous system, creating a state of sensitivity in which your entire brain is stimulated. This fully stimulated brain then integrates signals as they are received. The result is a crystal clarity in your perceptions, your thoughts, and your intuition. That's why Kundalini yoga is often called "the yoga of awareness."

When we apply the ancient skills and teachings of yoga through ongoing practice, we form a communion with ourselves and the soul growing inside us. Our outer and inner selves merge more completely, and we come to know the serene source of strength and compassion that is the very center of our beings.

It is always my deepest prayer that as you begin to use the technology of this wonderful science we call Kundalini yoga, you will see a real shift in your life toward greater well-being and happiness, and will be inspired to devote more of your time to these life-changing techniques, creating a more fulfilled life for yourself, your children, your family, and your world in the process. May this pregnancy spark your own lifelong exploration.

This book isn't a manual. It is not a "new, better, different" strategy for childbirth. It isn't about "managing" your pregnancy. Just as yoga is a practice of self-acceptance rather than an exercise program for self-improvement, the Kundalini yoga and meditations included here are meant to lead you back to what you already know inside you. The experience of having a child is complete unto itself. It needs only to be cherished for what it is.

I offer this book to you as a tool, in the knowledge that the ancient practices of the yogic tradition can ignite within you your own innate knowingness. One of the greatest challenges of pregnancy, and of being a parent, is that you can't look to anyone else for lessons on how to do it. You can find inspiration, you can learn techniques, but each child and each birth is as unique as a snowflake; no one is exactly like another.

For thousands upon thousands of years, no one read books on birthing, because there weren't any. Though they didn't know about due dates, they knew to count the waxing and waning of the moon. Above all, they knew very, very well how they *felt*. Each person on earth is the manifestation of eons of successful birthing. That ancient knowledge is in every woman's bones and stored in our very cells. In this book, you will hear the voices and the stories of many other women, in the timeless way that the wisdom surrounding birth, child-rearing, and caring for our precious bodies has been passed from generations of women for centuries.

Throughout this book I offer time-tested techniques, meditations, and exercises that will help you physically, mentally, and spiritually. Do as much as feels comfortable at first. You will find as you continue that you will be able to increase the length and duration as your strength and focus increases. I pass these teachings on from the depth of my heart as they have been passed to me in this Golden Chain of women who came before, each and all of them teachers, mothers, saints, warriors, leaders, and beloved. In their name I pray you have a healthy baby, a happy pregnancy, and that you are inspired to become a conscious parent who makes conscious choices.

What do I mean when I say "conscious"? It might be easier to explain what I don't mean. I am not talking about developing a new belief system. What it means to be conscious is to experience genuinely what is actually in front of you and to evaluate your life for the truth of what is really there, rather than through the "consensus reality" of what society, the media, our families, peers, whoever, tells us *should* be there, or what we *should* be doing, or what we *have* to do. Experience the world for yourself, and use your own intuition and intelligence to make choices.

We have a saying, "As a woman lives, so shall she birth." If you are living in calmness, radiance, joy, and good health, this is the atmosphere into which your baby will be born and grow. My first concern for you is to have a healthy baby, the second is to be as active and present a participant as you can be, and the third is to enjoy the process of bringing a new soul through you.

This book is your permission to laugh, to dance, to cry, and to reach beyond whatever you previously thought possible. This is also a time to question all that you have held to be true in the past about your relationships, your body, how you will birth, and how you will parent. Preparing for your life as a mother is like going through the heat of a forge, tempering the steel of your mind and strengthening your spirit. Seize the force of creation that whirls inside of you and never look back!

BLESSINGS,

GURMUKH

LOS ANGELES 2002

THE
FIRST
TRIMESTER

*. . . an opening to our
own minds, emotions,
and intuition, and
a deeper knowledge
of ourselves . . .*

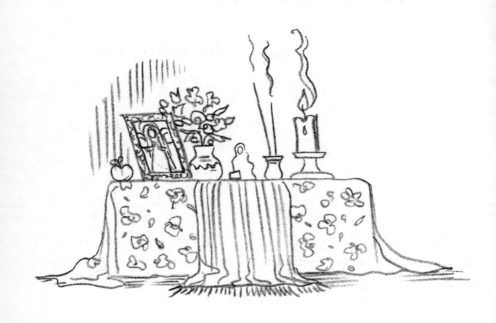

THE FIRST
STEP OF
THE JOURNEY

*"Not understanding
yourself is not
understanding
the Truth."*

— S O E N - S A

Y ou're pregnant? *Wahe Guru!* Which is to say, the experience of the Infinite Creator is so great it's beyond words.

I remember so well the dawning realization that I wasn't just late—I was actually going to have a baby. I would stand in line at the grocery store and wonder if
strangers could tell there was something wonderful happening inside me. In my
mind, it was the headline of every newspaper. When my husband and I married, we
didn't know if we could have children; he hadn't been able to have a child with his
first wife for eight years, and it had been twenty years for me. I wanted to sing from
the rooftops, "Hey, look everybody, I'm pregnant!"

Instead, I sang on the inside. In those first early days of pregnancy, it's best to
keep it a secret between you and your partner until you know for sure, until that
spark has fanned into a flame. Only let good vibrations go toward the energy it takes
to grow a soul. You don't want the energy of anyone who is jealous, or worried, or
just not "on your side" to be directed to you or the baby. The first three months are
like preparing the ground before the garden is planted. "I kept it as a delicious

secret," said a friend of mine of the first three months of her first pregnancy. "The experience was mine, all mine, to savor."

Years ago my teacher, Yogi Bhajan, gave us the perfect metaphor for understanding. "Life does not start in your womb on the first day of conception," he stated in the calm, heartfelt way that is the signature of a great teacher. "Look at the natural law. We build a house first, fix it up, then enter it. Nobody digs the ground for a foundation and then moves the furniture in!" Why would God be any different?

I know this is another example of how everything in nature is perfectly arranged and timed. The first one hundred and twenty days are given to us as a time to strengthen the foundation of our lives, in order for us to be prepared for the seismic shift that comes with having a child. That is true whether it is your first baby or your fifth, because each birth gives you a new opportunity to penetrate your understanding even more deeply and grow in your love and wisdom.

If you already have children, you know the truth of what I am about to tell you, and if you don't have children, just ask anybody who does: When you have a baby you will never act as if you are single again. Children are a bigger commitment than marriage, than a mortgage, than a career. So much attention is given to the last months of pregnancy and birth, but in some respects the first trimester might present the biggest challenge because it requires an adjustment within your psyche. Your definition of self changes from "I" to "we." To have a child is to undergo transformation.

This is not an understanding you can "think" your way into. You cannot birth intellectually. You birth sensually, intuitively, primally, and spiritually. You can't cram at the end—it takes nine months to unfold your consciousness. Pregnancy is a partnership of mother and child, and it takes almost ten months to build. Birth is a miraculous doorway that opens to our own mental, emotional, and intuitive growth, and a deeper knowledge, appreciation, and love of our bodies and ourselves.

Intellectual knowledge only becomes real wisdom when you experience it in your own heart and being. That requires discipline to act in a way that nourishes you and to surrender to a process that is greater than your individual self. Discipline means to be a disciple of your true self that lies within. It does not come from the outside, be it parent, church, teacher, whomever. That's why beginning a yoga and meditation practice now will reap big rewards. You give to the soul who chose you the gift of being as great as you can be so that you may shepherd him or her through this lifetime.

According to ancient teachings, souls don't just randomly reincarnate. There is a specific, divine plan. You, as parents, are a big part of that plan. Relax. Ultimately, a soul can never fail in its path to perfect realization. To succeed, the soul will come back as many times as necessary to fulfill its spiritual mission. I often return to India, my spiritual home, where there are a billion souls living in a land slightly larger than the size of Texas. It is the most unbelievable experience every time my family and I go. It moves me to see all these souls who have traveled across infinity to reincarnate in a land where there are so many, and such hard karma. So much spirit is present in these people because that is all most of them have.

Just as within the yogic tradition, the Jewish Kabbalists teach that our souls chose our parents, because only particular parents can teach a particular soul what it has to learn in this lifetime. There can be a number of reasons for the choice—past life relationships, or simply that the environment these parents can provide is conducive to the soul achieving its overall mission. Parents can teach by positive example, and sometimes by negative example. The process of parenting is about what the soul brings to you, and what you need to bring to that soul.

One concept of karma I like is that souls enter in a cluster, like constellations of stars. It has been said that we as souls make a contract before reincarnating regarding where, when, and how we will come back to very specific parents, sometimes through a petri dish or surrogate mothers or adoption. Each of us brings the other in, like bridges—I hold my arms out so someone else can come through me.

Though the soul is pure and complete, an expression of the universe, there is the subtle body, an energy force surrounding the soul, that carries the karma of the previous life. Your soul comes back with a destiny, a path to walk this lifetime, and you come back bringing gifts you have acquired—all of this is what we call karma. "As you sow so shall you reap," is how I like to think of it. A mother can actually purify the karma by her own devotion to living an awakened life *and thus change the destiny of this soul within.* That doesn't mean being perfect and doing everything by the book, it means living with compassion and awareness, which is your own innate nature as woman, as mother.

There is an old tale from India about a queen mother who had become pregnant. On the one hundred and twenty-fifth day she suddenly got very sick, and was told by an oracle that she had attracted the soul of a demon who would wreak havoc on the kingdom and make her life a living hell. Distraught, this queen went to the Raaj Guru, the royal spiritual guide, and began to weep.

"Oh my teacher, can you be kind to me and bless me?" she implored. "Whatever my karma is, so be it."

The teacher looked at her and said, "All is not lost. From this day forward, meditate on the name of God, and go out among your people and serve them selflessly, and practice the teachings of the ancient ways." So the queen left her palace and went out into the streets, cooking meals, washing dishes, and feeding the poor. When the day of her labor finally came, the boy was born smiling, with his hands peacefully pressed in a yogic *mudra* and an impression in his forehead at the Third Eye point, which is at the center of the brow between the eyes. The baby grew up not to be a demon, but a saint. The womb is where another human being, through her compassion and knowingness, can help change the destiny, or facilitate or uplift the destiny, of that soul inside her. This is our gift on the planet as women. This is the way we can change the world and bring peace to this planet.

I think about that tale every time the moms from my prenatal class come back after they have given birth to attend the postnatal classes. The faces of their babies! People arrive in a baby costume, there's no doubt. Some of these children look ancient. One little baby I held recently, if he had worn a tapered beard, would have inspired me to say, "Blessings to you, Old Sage!" Others look like Gerber babies. No two are ever identical, even if they are identical twins. That is why we need the time during pregnancy to become the kind of mother who has the intuitiveness to see who our babies really are and what they need.

Your journey to being that kind of mother begins now, even before you become pregnant, in fact. You will find it so much more delightful than zeroing in on only the medical, finite plane of pregnancy. Learning to meditate will attract all you are longing to understand. It will allow you to create a space in your mind amid the tests and technology and all the things swirling around you right now. From that space, you can enter your own knowing. Meditation means learning to watch the thousands of thoughts created by the mind and not judge them or be attached to one, just as we are not fixed on one drop of water as we observe the flow of a river. With practice, you will arrive at a clear and serene space inside you where you can begin to know your true nature.

MEDITATION MADE EASY

To begin meditation, choose a place that is clean, uncluttered, and quiet. Your body needs to be comfortably warm but not too hot (that can make you sleepy). It's best if you haven't eaten a full meal in two hours. Wear loose, light-colored, and natural-fiber clothing if possible, which will expand your body's aura or energy field by a foot and a half. That is your sacred space. Make sure you are barefoot because you want your feet to breathe. The feet contain seventy-two thousand nerve endings that stimulate the energy and health within your entire body. Sit on a rug or towel or even a pillow. A light blanket or shawl for covering your body and your head is also help-ful. If you reserve this covering only for that purpose, it will come to contain a cer-tain meditative vibration that you will find relaxing just by putting it on.

Now you are ready for the first and most basic yogic posture, **Easy Pose**:

- Sitting on the mat, fold your right leg and place it under the left knee, then bend the left leg and place the foot under the right knee.
- You may sit with a folded blanket or pillow under the back part of your but-tocks to help support your back. If for some reason you can't sit comfortably

on the floor, sit in a straight-backed chair to keep your posture straight. Or, sit on the floor with your legs straight out and your back against a wall. Keep your back as straight as possible.

• Imagine a string is attached to your head, pulling it up to the ceiling, making sure to tuck your chin slightly to lengthen your spine.

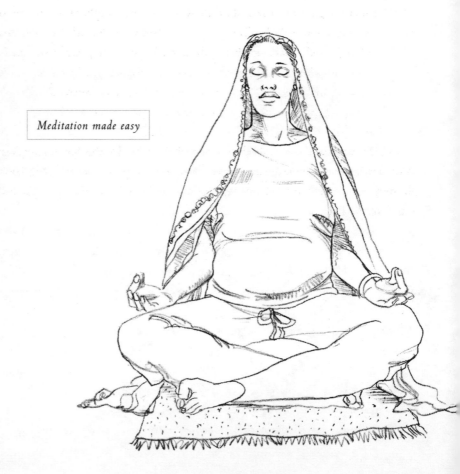

Meditation made easy

- Relax your shoulders and drop them down away from your ears.
- Close your eyes and roll them up as if you are looking at the middle of your forehead. This is the Third Eye point, source of your intuition. If at first this is challenging, begin by simply rolling your eyes upward.
- Relax into the position and let your breath flow deeply into your body. Breathe from your baby's home. Relax your hands onto your knees, palms facing up. Press your index fingers and thumbs firmly together. This is called *gyan mudra*, and creates wisdom.
- Inhale through your nose and exhale through your mouth. Hear the sound "Sat" on the inhale, "Nam" on the exhale. The sound "Sat" rhymes with the word "lot," and "Nam" rhymes with "mom." "Sat Nam" means "Truth Is My Identity." I encourage you to use these sounds, because the yogic science of *naad*, which is the repeating of certain syllables, was created to open up and stimulate subtle nerve centers in your body to enhance well-being.

Make sure the inhale and exhale are equal in length. Do this for eleven minutes. Although meditation will benefit you at any point in your day, it is especially good in the morning as a way to center yourself for the day ahead, and before going to bed at night to help you relax fully.

PREGNANCY
AS A LIVING
PRAYER

$2 + 2 = 5.$

—YOGI BHAJAN

Whenever I see homeless people, I think, Where are their mothers? If a mother forever prays for her children, they will always be guided, guarded, and protected. The ultimate extreme is when a mother stops and says, "Forget it, this child is no good" or "I give up on him" or just throws her hands up in disgust—that creates all those lost people you see on the street. At the same time, if a mother is always fearful of her children's well-being, from in utero to infant to adult, that child will undoubtedly be affected by that fear and become fearful also. On the other hand, when a mother is joyful, strong, disciplined in her well-being and prayerful, so her children will be.

God means:

G for Generator
O for Organizer
D for Deliverer

Everything moves by God. Seeing this, feeling this, and experiencing this realm of consciousness in all that is around us is called living prayer. Whenever your heart pours into prayer, every heartbeat creates a miracle. The power of mankind is in our prayer. This is why real change and real peace can only come through prayer. The brilliant Irish poet John O'Donohue reminds us that prayer is never wasted: "It always brings transformation. . . . Prayer refines you so that you may become worthy of your possibility and destiny."

How do we pray? Concentrate and project outward. My teacher once said that prayer is a telephone call through the universal exchange. "If the current is strong, though the distance is long, it will be heard at the other end. Help will come."

A mother's prayer holds the sacred space for her child, a mother's prayer holds the world. Nothing is as profound nor as powerful as a mother who prays. I was moved to tears by this story one student told: After a forest fire in Yellowstone, a ranger found a bird literally petrified in ashes, perched on the ground next to the base of a tree. Struck by the eerie sight, he took a stick and tipped the bird over. Three tiny chicks scurried from under the dead mother's wings. The loving mother bird, who must have been keenly aware of the impending disaster, carried her babies to the base of the tree and gathered them under her wings to protect them from the toxic smoke. She could have flown to safety, but did not. When the blaze arrived and the heat scorched her body, she stayed steadfast. Because she was willing to die, those chicks lived under the cover of her wings. What a reminder of the boundlessness and fierce belief in the future we as mothers are capable of expressing.

A soul chooses the mother in whose womb it will grow and be nurtured. Yogi Bhajan has said that "from the beginning of life to its end it is only a mother who can vibrate for her child and change his destiny. It is only the mother whose vibrations and prayers can affect like an arc beam, and the child's written destiny only she can wipe out and rewrite."

There is a Sikh story about how the prayer of a mother has the power to reverse even death itself. The story goes that a woman went to a sage and asked for a child. The sage said, "So be it," and gave her the mantra "Siri Akaal," which means "great undying." She soon gave birth to a beautiful child. One day while working in the field, she strayed from the baby as she worked. Unbeknown to her, a cobra came and bit the child, who soon died of the venom. When the mother came back, she refused to accept his death. She wanted two things: her son back among the living and the cobra dead. So she sat down and chanted this mantra. It was so powerful when spoken by the mother that the cobra reversed his action, and the child started to breathe once more. Then, the cobra asked forgiveness, but that wasn't so easy. He was, after all, dealing with a mother who had vengeance on her mind. She said, "No. You took the life of my child, and you will not live to take the life of any child again." To save his skin, the cobra vowed that no saintly child would ever again be bitten by a cobra. One of our saints, Guru Nanak, slept one day as a baby with his face in the sun. A cobra came and made shade to acknowledge the vow that a divine child would never suffer from that snake again.

My teacher has said, "Once you give birth to a child, give him the highest gift: prayer." My daughter goes to school in India nine months of the year. She is just completing her twelfth year in a school our dharma organization built in the countryside of northern India for children of all faiths. She is eighteen now, and this is her last year of school in India. No matter where she is, I never feel she is far from me. While I was pregnant with her, I awoke at three-thirty every morning to do *sadhana*, our morning prayers. In those nine months, we developed a communication that is stronger than any words, an invisible link that bonds us even now. She is always with me. Whenever I want to talk to her, to be close and to tell her how very much I love her, I shut my eyes and pray. Across thousands of miles I know she hears me, as I hear her when she prays.

CREATING A SACRED SPACE

Make an altar in your home. Start simple. I used to take a cardboard box, turn it upside down, and cover it with a nice, clean cloth, flowers, candles, and pictures of my loved ones, and there it was. I would sit on a little rug in front of it and begin my morning practice. Today, every room in my house has an altar, to the divine mother, to life, to God, and I am forever decorating them.

Altars take you back to your source, to what is really essential. An altar can be an earthly extension of your spirit. To sit in the same place every day for your yoga and meditation is good, because that space starts to take on the meditative energy you create. It will actually start to feel different from the rest of your home. Any quiet place is fine, like the corner of your bedroom. We once had a student who converted her second bathroom into a little meditation room; I took a small closet in my house and decorated it like a temple, so I can have one place where I can close the door and everyone will know not to disturb me because I am meditating.

Extend your being, and your baby's, onto an altar and see how it feels. Let the altar "alter" your spirits! When you leave for the day you will take this altar with you in your heart.

To relax at your altar, come sitting into Easy Pose, with your hands pressed together at the center of your chest.

Creating a sacred space

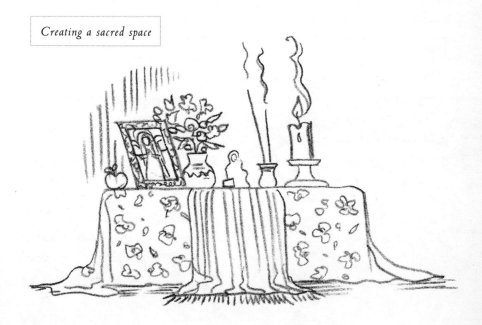

- Repeat the sounds "Ong Namo Guru Dev Namo" three times. The words mean: "I am bowing to that creative wisdom inside myself." It might be strange for you at first to say these words if you have never used a mantra before. If you are too uncomfortable, you can say, "I bow to that creative all knowingness that is written in my very being." These ancient sounds will take you from outside yourself and from all the information that bombards you throughout the day to the inside of you, which is quiet, empty, and beyond the mere intellect. Meditation will give you clarity and awareness if you have a strong faith already.
- Inhale deeply through your nose, and chant like singing. Repeat this at least three times, or do as many as eleven or twenty-six to reach a state of equanimity.

After you have established an area in your home where you can be quiet and feel undisturbed, add this meditation when you are ready:

MEDITATION FOR INFINITE CONNECTION

- Still sitting in Easy Pose, bring your arms forward and cup your hands together with the pinkie fingers touching, six inches in front of your heart center.
- Pull your spine straighter as you sit.
- Gently lower your eyes and softly focus them in front of you, and feel the supreme energy coming down from the heavens and merging with the flow of life inside you.
- Do this for three minutes, inhaling and exhaling through your nose, or as long as you are comfortable, and end with a deep inhale and exhale. Relax.

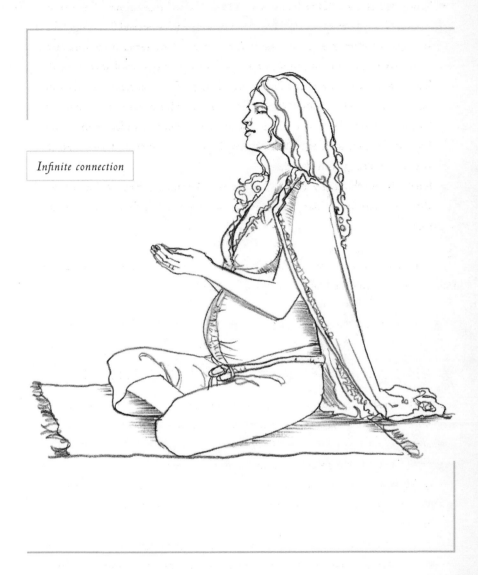

Infinite connection

BOUNTIFUL,
BEAUTIFUL,
BLISSFUL

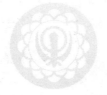

"... she shall be the
mother of nations."

—GENESIS 17:16

The essence of woman is bountiful, beautiful, and blissful. This pregnancy is a gift to free you in the largest sense by revealing your true nature. The teaching of Kundalini yoga is that a woman comes to know and love herself, radiance shines through to the outside, and we call her beautiful. As she grows to be compassionate not only of others but of herself, we call her bountiful. Finally, as she comes to experience the vastness of who she is and of what she is capable, we call her blissful.

Everything in the physical world comes though the *yoni*, the womb of the female, creative force of the universe. It is amazing when you think about it. I remember walking down a street in Los Angeles when I found out I was pregnant, seeing the faces of the people who passed me as if I was seeing humankind for the first time. There were young and old, men, women, teenagers, toddlers, infants, big people, small people, some with round eyes, some with slanted eyes, some with eyes that look you up and down as you pass, ones with brown skin the shade of walnuts, smooth black skin, some so white it seemed the sun would just reflect right off them! Each of them was a marvel to me. I put my arms around my middle and thought of the cells dividing and dividing and dividing, even in that moment as I walked down the street. It hit me that each of these human beings I was seeing got here the very same way: one sperm, one egg, and a woman who carried them in her body. It's an everyday occurrence, but when it's happening to you it seems the most extraordinary event on the planet.

Our babies are created in the only viable place in our bodies they could come from: the center, the point from which our *chi*, or life energy, radiates. The navel represents the third chakra, the fundamental element of commitment. Our babies feed on this energy, and are sustained by it, becoming the sun, the center of the universe, the center of their mothers. The arrangement could not be more perfect.

Some of you might be reading this and think, "Yes, I know exactly what she means." Others of you will roll your eyes and say, "What is she talking about? My body is being invaded by an alien, and I don't like it!" Believe me, even if you don't feel it, you can. A lot of it has to do with getting back in touch—or getting in touch for the very first time—with yourself, with your feelings, with your body. You'll be able to rely on that self-knowledge again and again.

One summer at our ashram in New Mexico, we women gathered before dawn each morning on a grassy knoll facing east as the sun crept out of the horizon to shed its gold on the broad range of the Sangre de Cristo Mountains. If you have ever sat in the middle of a New Mexico sunrise, you know why it's called the Land of Enchantment. The air is sweet with the scent of piñon, the sky so close and clear it's as if you could just reach up into it and come away with a handful of blue. And so we would sit for thirty-one minutes with our right hand straight forward, palm facing down, reaching for the horizon at sixty degrees. The left hand would be at the knee in *gyan mudra*, thumb pressed to index finger and the other fingers kept straight. In unison we would recite this mantra so that we might know and feel in every fiber of our being that we are the creative force of the universe:

I am the light of my soul
I am bountiful
I am beautiful
I am bliss
I am, I AM

These are simple words, but the effect they have is powerful when we take them to heart and accept them as the truth of who we are.

As you go through your pregnancy, you'll hear a lot about "childbirth preparation." The challenge with any preparation technique is that it can make birth seem more predictable than it is. By stressing techniques that manage pain, we get the implied message that if we're just diligent enough, if we are good students and pass our childbirth education classes with an "A," we can control the situation when it comes time for the baby to be born. The fact is, labor is unpredictable and resists all of our best-laid plans to control it. Often I'll have women seek out our classes for their second pregnancies, because they want to rethink their approach—the common refrain I always hear is, "I had no idea it would be like *that!*" So many of us go into labor ill-prepared for the overwhelming, powerful sensations we experience. And then what does our mind tell us to do? Panic. "Give me that epidural NOW!"

How can we not panic? Begin to cultivate a balanced state of being. Yoga and meditation keeps your body aligned, keeps you strong physically and mentally, and balances your glandular system, your brain, your circulatory system, and your hormones, and allows your spirit to rise. With yoga we can develop a sense of equanimity that takes us not only through our pregnancy but into the next chapter of our life—mothering.

HONORING YOUR WOMANHOOD

Do the Bountiful, Beautiful meditation given above. If you can't be outdoors, find a quiet place indoors where you won't be disturbed, light a candle and sit facing east, where each new day is born. Announce to yourself, to your baby, your creator, and the world that you are the light of the soul! Listen to yourself. Speak softly, loudly, or in a whisper—however the spirit moves you. Sit for three to eleven minutes. Challenge yourself to keep your arm up the entire time.

I am the light of my soul
I am bountiful
I am beautiful
I am bliss
I am, I AM

Honoring your womanhood

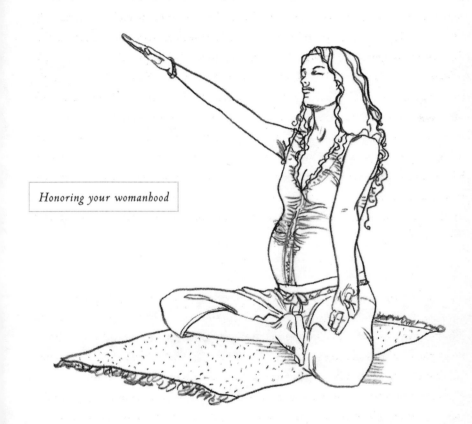

THE
EMOTIONAL
ABYSS

inda came into class looking as if she had been put through the spin cycle of the washing machine. Her face was the color of ashes, and her shoulders slumped dejectedly. I wasn't five minutes into teaching when she sprang up from her yoga mat, hand over her mouth, and made a run to the restroom. "I thought 'morning' sickness was only in the morning," she lamented after class. "Nobody told me it could be morning, mid-morning, noon, afternoon, evening, and sometimes at night sickness."

Linda was well into what I call The Abyss, that stretch of time, almost always just in the first trimester of pregnancy, that is sometimes spent in sickness, exhaustion, and often confusion. Sickness because you're nauseated and woozy, as if you're on a small boat in a rough sea and you can't get off; exhaustion because the changes in your body are so big; confusion because the sensation is disorienting, and you think it will never end. Not every woman experiences these symptoms, but for those of us who do, it can be a real challenge.

As in planting, the seed is far under the soil right now. No sunlight needed yet, just water and time. Sometimes we feel that everything is happening so deep within us. I remember it as a twilight zone. I wasn't me anymore, and I wasn't my future as a mother. I was in an in-between land, waiting for the hidden seed to pop out of darkness into the light. For me, this time was more difficult than giving birth. I felt sick, out of control, and many times anxious, as if I had a pinball machine inside me that was being played twenty-four hours a day. I would have loved a book like this or a pregnancy yoga class, or just someone to laugh with and say, "I'm glad I'm not the only one who's feeling crazy!" Many times in my class new mothers come up at the end for a hug, their eyes brimming with tears. In fact, most eyes fill with water after we sing our closing song. The heart opens, the spirit joins with others, and in that way, fear takes a back seat!

During a hot summer in New Mexico in 1985, I was at Ladies Camp, a special retreat we have had for women every summer for the last thirty years. Women come from all over the world to be together, study yoga, hike, and swim. We study the ancient teachings on women and our essence and power with Yogi Bhajan. We leave the men and children at home. Our Sikh teachings tell us women should come together, removing themselves from their routine and taking time to relax, get back to the rhythm of nature, laugh, and tend to themselves. This retreat recharges us for the entire year so that we'll be well and happy when we return home.

Off I went for my first summer after marriage to lead aerobics classes every morning at 9 A.M. Back then, the camp went for a full six weeks; I was camping in a tent with my best friend, who by the age of twenty-four already had four children. Here was old me at forty-two, with major morning sickness. Every morning I would tell my friend, "I'm sick—go tell them I can't teach. Make something up!" No one at camp knew about my pregnancy except the two of us. But every morning, in her kind but insistent way, she would say, "Go teach and you'll feel better." So I would drag myself—usually crying and so mad at her for ordering me to do something I didn't feel like doing—to the recreation hall and teach. By the time class ended, I always felt better. That was how I learned that moving and being with others helps morning sickness and tiredness. God bless my friend for teaching me that lesson—she was my guardian angel, and still is in so many ways.

In teaching pregnant women all these years, I've noticed women have a tendency to think, "I am pregnant, therefore I will have morning sickness, heartburn, my back will hurt, I will have shooting pains down my legs, I will feel like there is not enough room in my body for me and the baby"—all the old wives' tales and everything they have seen and heard from friends who have gone before them into motherhood. To all that I say, "No." Feeling bad does not have to be the way you spend your pregnancy—just like feeling bad all the time in your life is unnecessary. True, some women suffer and go through more than others when they're expecting. Maybe your diet needs adjusting, or maybe you need to move in a way that will stimulate your body's own healing energy; or just talk to someone. There are ways through almost everything in pregnancy so that you may flow and grow.

Yogis know that ginger root tea can help regulate the wild flux of hormones in these early stages, support your nervous system, and cleanse your liver. I recommend making the tea yourself from fresh ingredients—it's just as easy as dunking a teabag: Finely chop about 1 inch of fresh ginger root (found at most grocery stores) and add it to 1 cup water. Let it boil for five minutes, then add a little honey, milk (soy or regular) or a squish of lemon. Drink up! It's yummy.

Remember, whatever you're feeling, it is only temporary in the scheme of things. During the first three months of pregnancy, you can feel like you're a little gopher burrowed underground in your own little world. Usually around the third, into the fourth, month, the sun starts to shine down that hole you're in, and the world starts to look brighter. One day, you will look out of your gopher hole, sniff the air, and feel the sunshine and say, "Wow! There is a world out there after all!"

During her first pregnancy, a student, Elizabeth, developed a particularly beautiful point of view we can all learn from: "I believe that the child chooses us, and we must honor that. Being a mother, having my husband supporting me, is a privilege I can't take for granted. When I can remember to come from that space, I act completely differently. When I come from some other space, like 'Why is this happening to me? It's not fair,' that's when I start to feel tired and cranky." *Gratitude helps so much.*

Terrific perspectives on this came to me from a stately older woman, an editor at a magazine. She had given birth to two sons, now grown to be handsome men. "I found everything about pregnancy to be somewhat amusing, like the flip-flop of my stomach when I got within a foot of food," she recalled. "I learned to love and embrace every discomfort and every comfort—everything, because tomorrow it will be gone. Tomorrow, it will be something else."

EXERCISE FOR EMOTIONAL BALANCE

This exercise energizes by building your electromagnetic field, and improves the balance in the hemispheres of your brain so that your whole body can adjust itself:

- In Easy Pose, stretch your arms up above your ears with the palms facing each other stretching to the sky. The fingers are side by side but the thumbs are separate. Keep your arms and palms stiff as steel, reaching high the entire time.
- Begin to move the arms back and forth like you are fanning your head, six to nine inches out, and then back in. Your eyes are closed and rolled upward. Move powerfully for at least three minutes, working up to seven minutes.

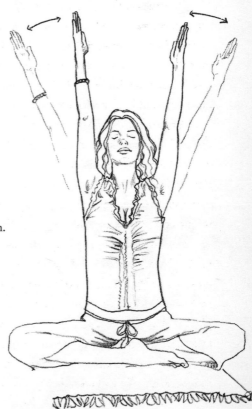

Emotional balance

MORNING
SICKNESS

Yes, food can be a challenge right now. A drop in your blood glucose levels caused by the added work your body is doing to create a baby is enough to make you feel fatigued, irritable, and emotional. Your sense of smell is heightened, and cooking might be the last thing you can imagine doing. Just the smell of coffee might be enough to make you run for the bathroom.

Nurse midwife Davi Kaur Khalsa, my partner in the childbirth education program we offer at Golden Bridge, always recommends that expectant moms eat something every two hours, preferably a little bit of protein and a vegetable or fruit, but even plain pasta is fine if that's all you can get down and *keep* down! For right now, just get what you can and don't get caught in a world of "shoulds"—"I should be doing this," "I should be doing that...." The baby gets what the baby needs, which is your body, Mommy. That's okay. You will regain yourself.

Eat as many whole, live, and organic foods as you possibly can. Sometimes you can start to feel better through diet alone, because your body's glucose levels stabilize when you start to eat regularly at two-hour intervals. Tell your partners I said this: If the pregnant woman you are with is cranky and feeling sick, don't tell her to eat something. Prepare something that appeals to her, and then feed it to her!

A friend of mine who grew up in a large Italian family once told me jokingly that "the family that eats together, stays together." In her case the parents and the kids and the cousins and grandparents all got together at least once a week for a great home-cooked Italian meal. Today, scientists tell us that there's something to that: When we sit down to eat with each other, we look into each other's eyes, which actually stimulates the release of the "love" hormone oxytocin, the same hormone that contracts the uterus during birth, that gives us the universal sense of "falling in love," that even bonds a mother to her baby. So pull up a chair, and eat together!

Make a commitment never to leave the house without a snack bag full of healthy goodies—no white sugar, no white flour. Make sure there is a variety, because you never know what's going to appeal to you. Try raisins, almonds, fruit, crackers, or soy nuts. Make sure to pack enough protein! Get a nice little basket or cloth bag for your goodies, and a water bottle you can easily fill to keep hydrated.

GOOD-BYE TO QUEASINESS

Walk for a half hour, and as you walk press the thumbs of both hands to each of the fingertips in the following order: thumb to index, thumb to middle finger, thumb to ring finger, thumb to pinkie. Each of these are actually *mudras* to provide specific benefits:

- Thumb to index finger is *gyan mudra* for knowledge
- Thumb to middle finger *is shuni mudra* for wisdom, intelligence, and patience
- Thumb to ring finger is *surya mudra* for vitality
- Thumb to pinkie is *bhudi mudra* for the ability to communicate well

Verbally or mentally chant in a monotone the syllables Sa-Ta-Na-Ma, one syllable to each finger. Continue, starting each round with the index finger and ending with the pinkie. If it helps, do it every day.

Walking balances the brain, hormones, and the glandular and nervous systems. Walk with a friend or your partner if you can. We say up to five miles a day at a steady, comfortable pace is good, but gauge yourself. If after you finish your walk you feel exhausted and need more than two hours of sleep to recover, reassess. Are you getting a full night's sleep and keeping hydrated? If you are and still felt exhausted after exercise, then you might be overdoing it. Ease up! Be observant and watch how you're doing, especially if you're a "Type A" personality.

Good-bye to queasiness

THE
IMPORTANCE
OF BREATH

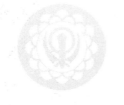

*"Breath is
the kiss of God."*

—YOGI BHAJAN

As you breathe and as you move, so will your baby throughout his life. The soul inside you is testing the climate upon the earth where he will walk. What he learns in the womb, a baby will live as an adult. Think about baby ducks—they walk and talk just like their mamas!

In yogic terms, the life force is named *prana*, which comes to us through breath. The ancient Greeks knew this; in fact the root of the word spirit is taken from the ancient Greek word for breath. *Yama* means control. *Pranayama*, the term we use in yoga, means directing the current of this vital energy to light your body to its most luminous. Allowing yourself to take in enough breath is the first thing you need to do, but it is often the last thing we remember. Breath relaxes. It also gives you clarity and cool-headedness, because it brings oxygen and nitrogen to the brain cells and pumps spinal fluid to the brain. It prevents the buildup of toxins in the lungs, and as the lung capacity expands, your pituitary gland, regulator of all the hormones in your body, becomes stimulated.

Sometimes when mothers come to Golden Bridge for the childbirth education program, they are expecting to learn a new pattern of breathing, like learning a workout routine! We say, breathing is *voluntary, not forced*. You don't need to learn complicated techniques. You just need to slow it down and make it more even. It is not about some rigid technique that takes you out of the experience of the moment you are living *right now*, it is about getting in touch with your natural breath *right now*.

More effective than learning a technique is to consider that breath is a path that will lead to focusing your mind on a visualization, or to creating your own mantra, words that encourage you to let your spirit do what it naturally is drawn to do. You want to get to the meditative mind that is all-expansive, not the "mental" mind, the bean counter mind, the mind that keeps schedules and makes judgments and gets scared! Breath is the axis between our earthly selves and the subtle, transcendent realms.

BREATHING BETTER EXERCISE

The oxygen-carrying capacity of your body increases during pregnancy, which is one of the reasons you can sometimes feel out of breath when you are pregnant. Yoga bolsters your circulatory system and gently stimulates all your organs so they can do their optimal job.

- First, stand erect. Open a hardcover book as if you are reading it, and press the lower edge against your navel three fingers' width below your belly button.
- As you inhale, your belly pushes the book away from your body. As you exhale, the book glides back toward your spine as the belly empties of air. If you let your stomach muscles relax completely as you inhale, your diaphragm will open, your lungs will fill to their capacity—maybe for the first time in years.

Now you are breathing as God intended you to breathe. Doing this, your blood becomes more highly oxygenated, which will fuel all your organs, including the nerve cells in your brain, so you will begin to think more clearly.

Once you have got the hang of it, close your eyes, focus at your Third Eye point. Inhale the sound Sat, exhale Nam. Do this for at least five minutes, up to as long as you like. It works whether you are preparing for pregnancy or in your last trimester. Babies love it for the calming effect it creates in the waters they live within.

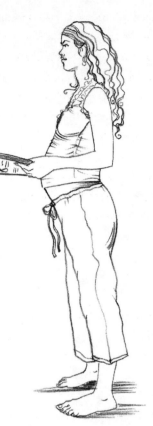

Breathing better exercise

HEALING
OLD WOUNDS

"Your soul longs to draw
you into love for
yourself. When you
enter your soul's
affection, the torment
in your life ceases."

—JOHN O'DONOHUE,
ETERNAL ECHOES

I am thinking of Sarah, whom I noticed in one of my classes. She sat near the back, her body seemed swallowed by a huge black T-shirt that could have doubled as a tent. I noticed her because she kept getting up to leave the room. At first I thought she was just feeling ill, then my intuition told me, No, she feels uncomfortable about her pregnancy and wants to avoid the emotions that are stirred by this yoga. Even though one part of her wants to do the exercises and meditations for the good of the baby, another part of her wants to hide and pretend she's not pregnant at all.

Talking to her confirmed this. "Pregnancy is embarrassing," Sarah told me. I encouraged her to keep coming to class, and slowly she revealed her life story: She had suffered three earlier miscarriages, and couldn't shake the belief that something was wrong with her, that her body wasn't "good enough." Even in her fourth pregnancy, when there was every indication she would carry to term, the feeling that her body wasn't an able vessel to carry a child would not go away. She was convinced that people looking at her pregnant form would sense this. I gave her this meditation to do each morning to remind herself of the truth: that she is whole and complete, and qualified to be a mother. For three minutes each day, Sarah found a quiet place, placed her left hand over her right hand and put them to her heart, shut her eyes and rolled them to the Third Eye point and repeated:

Happy am I
Healthy am I
Holy am I

I told her, when doubt set in anytime throughout the day, to put her hands to her heart and repeat this to herself silently or out loud until she felt centered and strong again.

Sarah gave birth to a chubby, gleeful baby boy. When she looked into his bright blue eyes, she told me, they seemed like the most precious jewels in the world to her. "But Sarah," I said, "your son's eyes are exactly your own. The same color, the same shape!" By seeing the perfection in the child her body had created, she began to see her own completeness as a human.

Another student had had an abortion when she was a teenager. Now that she was pregnant, she was troubled by thoughts of that first experience of pregnancy when she was a frightened young girl. It wasn't that she had a philosophical change of heart. She believed with all her heart in her right to make decisions in her own body, and she believed too that a soul doesn't enter the body until the one hundred and twentieth day after conception. What she came to realize is that some part of her had never pardoned that younger self for not mentally or emotionally being equipped to be a mother at that time. A part of her also had never mourned the loss of what could have been. So she wrote this letter:

Dear One,

I am sorry I wasn't able to be your mother back then. I was only fifteen and didn't know who I was or why I did the things I did. I had to have time to learn. I love you, and bless you on your journey.

It doesn't matter what your experience of pregnancy has been before this pregnancy. Even a painful experience carries the seeds of what will, with time, bloom into something lovely. Every experience we go through is something our own soul needs for its development. To grow in this experience of pregnancy, you need to explore yourself.

Start by digging into your belief system. Your wants and your wishes are one thing, but what is it that you really *know to be true*? Identifying that takes work, it takes sitting with yourself. How are your eyes seeing the world? What is your perception of birth? Of your doctor or midwife? Of spirituality, of the union between a fetus and your heart, or your union of your husband and yourself? We tend to give a cursory statement and just say, "This is how I feel." That is a rote answer. I have done it myself a thousand times. Knowing who you are and what you hold to be true takes time. Take each belief out of the box. Examine it, try it on again, check the seams—will it hold up? If something doesn't work—an attitude, a word, a description, an assumption—trim it off. Don't spend time punishing yourself about anything. In our society now we tend to be very psychologically aware and want to analyze ourselves, blaming ourselves—"Why did I think that? Stupid me!"—or interpret our past. Just release it and move on. Say, "This doesn't work," and shift. When I look back on my life, I could cry, I could get caught up in feelings of being immensely guilty, hurt, betrayed, you name it. Instead, all I feel is blessed, so blessed because all those life experiences made me the "me" I am today.

Sometimes we don't even realize how subtly dark and negative we are about our lives. We don't realize we are creating a world without the possibility of power. It is our choice to opt for light and the truth of our heart. I tell my students, misery is a choice you can always count on, it's always there as an option. Where are you going to stand in this process of becoming a mother? What you discover you can then take into every part of your life, but you have to make the discovery for yourself. No one can give it to you. I can't give it to you. Your doctor can't give it to you. Your husband can't give it to you. In fact, be suspicious of anyone who tells you he *can* give it to you! That opening inside yourself must come from you.

Know too that choosing to be positive is a process, something you do over and over again. It's not as if you will reach a point at which you will say, "Okay, now I'm fixed, now I will never know pain or anger or confusion." It is the doing over and over again. It is called a living "practice."

Childbirth is an ideal place to start to see the quality of the conversation you have with yourself.

MEDITATION FOR SELF-LOVE AND ACCEPTANCE

In practicing Kundalini, we are constantly creating the inner unity, the *yoga* of our individual self with the Infinite Self. For this meditation you will need a piece of fruit, any kind you like. The fruit will be charged with all of your self-love and acceptance, and then you will eat it, in effect giving back to yourself.

- Now, sit in Easy Pose with your left hand stretched straight out in front of you holding the fruit.
- Hold your opposite hand about four inches above the fruit. Keep your arms straight and your eyes closed.
- Concentrate on connecting the navel point to the fruit, as if you are taking the *prana*, or life force energy, and blessing the fruit. Keep going!
- After nine minutes, hold the fruit with both hands right at your navel point, and breathe long and deeply for two minutes.
- Then, with the fruit still at your navel, inhale as deeply as you can and then

lengthen the exhale out for as long as you can. Be conscious of this rhythm and continue for seven minutes.

• End by pressing the fruit against your navel—be careful not to squash it!—and press your tongue to your upper palate. Exhale, and then eat your fruit!

Self-love and acceptance

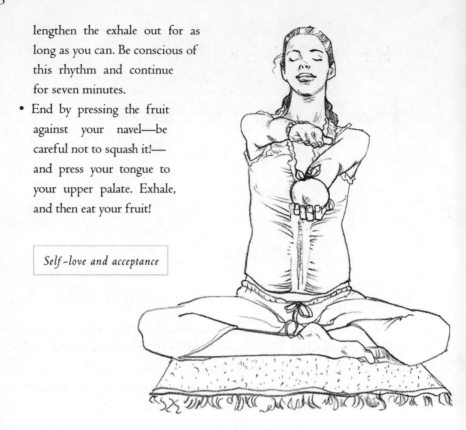

This is a great meditation to do for ninety days. This may seem like an impossibly long time for you, although you may surprise yourself. Start out with three minutes in each position if you like. In any case, the posture will put you through discomfort—it does for me, too! Keep up!

REMEMBERING
YOUR OWN
BIRTH

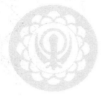

*"Know the mother
that you may
know the child."*

—QUAN YIN,
BUDDHIST GODDESS
OF COMPASSION

While I was pregnant with Wa, I never had a fear of labor. Instead, I was very afraid she would not be all right. At first I thought it was just the residual fear left over from the death of my first child. My mother was still alive while I was pregnant, and I spoke to her about that fear. "Oh, I worried while I was pregnant with you, too. A few weeks after you were born, that was the scariest time for me. Almost everything you ate you threw up," she commiserated. "You were basically starving to death. When you were only six weeks, we had to rush you to the hospital in Chicago twenty-three miles through a blizzard, and they performed surgery on you that night. They opened your pyloric valve that closed off to your stomach, so you could finally keep food down." They told my mother I would never be normal— they got that right! The doctors said it was a hereditary condition called plyoric stenosis that can happen during the first six weeks of a baby's life.

It was as if a lightbulb went off in my head. Of course! Not only was I carrying the fear from my own experience, but from my mother's as well. She must have been terrified that she could not do anything to make me better, almost sixty years ago before so many advances in medicine had been made. My own feelings of powerlessness and fear started to make more sense. Once I could see where they were rooted, I could begin to unearth them like weeds, to make room for new, positive feelings.

What makes us what we are today is what happened in the womb and in the first three years of life. For each month of pregnancy, you actually relive on a deep, emotional level your own time in the womb. Interview your own mother if possible to find out what she was thinking and feeling when she carried you. If your mother is no longer living, or you don't know your birth mother because you were adopted, hypnotherapy can be a tool to unlock that door, because somewhere in our cellular memory we have that knowledge. In fact, hypnotherapy, like meditation, can be incredibly healing.

One of our students, Camilia, reported that she had the most awesome feelings when she thought of delivering her child. Literally, she felt giddy and happy! Where did that feeling come from? Well, when she talked to her mother, her mother said she danced all through her pregnancy. Even while she was in labor, she had the strongest urge to dance. In the middle of the delivery room she insisted on getting up and doing a kooky belly dance. Imagining the picture of her mother in a hospital gown, dancing like a temple goddess, just cracked her up with laughter every time Camilia thought about it. Whenever she needed a pick-me-up, she too danced—and she also had a beautiful birth.

A friend of mine was so enriched by learning the details of her birth from her mother that she has made it a family ritual to tell the story of her children's birth every year on their birthday as a way to honor the event. The kids love it! If she forgets to do it, they remind her. Every year until my mother died several years ago at the age of ninety-three, she told the story of my birth in a birthday card, beginning with, "It was a cold winter night, and we drove through the snow to Chicago...." As I would read the cards each year, I could swear I almost felt the snow on my cheeks between the tears.

Not all of us, unfortunately, have such good or loving experiences of our family. Pregnancy can also be a time when old fears and angers against our parents surface very strongly. Some of us vow never to be like our parents, especially if we suffered any kind of abuse or neglect. This is a hard truth to hear: Even though we may feel completely justified in our anger and sorrow, holding on to it only serves to weaken us. It takes up psychic energy that holds us back from creating new, better experiences. Begin the process of healing your family history now while you are creating the new life that will come into this world.

In the Bible's Old Testament, the commandment does not obligate us to love our parents, but to honor them. To honor our parents means to acknowledge them as people of tremendous worth in our life's pilgrimage. Directly or indirectly, they put the fire behind your passion to grow toward your spiritual advancement. Honoring them is the most dignified endeavor of your life.

One of our students, a writer, told me she had always harbored a deep resentment and hatred for the man who fathered her, because he left her mother before she could tell him she was pregnant. Now that she was pregnant with her own son, she wanted to let go of that feeling. She didn't want to carry a dark anger toward men, to her very own son, or to her husband. Since she had no way of getting in touch with the man who had fathered her, she wrote this letter as a way of healing the wound. She shares it with us in the hope that we all can move beyond whatever pain we carry:

Dear Julio,

You are my father. That might come as a surprise to you. Come to think of it, I have no direct evidence you would know that, during the long winter of 1961 on your visit to the United States, you sired a child with that red-headed nursing student you dated.

This is what I know about you: your name, the town you told my mother you were from in Spain, that you wore linen shirts, and that you said my mother's name with a thick accent, "Patri-cia." She loved the sound of it on your tongue. You were young, she said. Younger, I realize, than I am now.

All that remains of you here is me, and five color photos from the night my mother cooked you your one Thanksgiving dinner here in America, cranberry sauce and giblet gravy, the works. From the five photos, I can see I have a vague resemblance to you in the curve of my nose and the straight shot of my eyebrows. After I learned about you, I used to sit in my mom's room and study those five pictures as if clues were written on them in invisible ink. I found evidence for why you would think my mother was good enough to sleep with but not to talk to after the fact, and why you would return letters containing my baby picture unopened: You hunched your shoulders—a sure sign of weakness. You wore a pullover sweater vest, testament to your petit bourgeois sensibilities. I came to see yours as the face of an otherwise nameless plague, the plague of men who deny their responsibility in the procreation process and have the luxury of denying that which does not suit them.

Julio, I want to ask your forgiveness for that. I know nothing about you or your circumstance or why or how you made the choices you did. I have grown into a person who has made my own mistakes and hurt a great many people in the process, and I have no right or authority to judge anyone, least of all you. I need to thank you for your part in creating me. In fact, deep down, when I was young and felt doomed by my mother's family history of alcoholism and poverty, I would think about your unknown blood in my veins and believe it was my salvation. Like Superman's cape, your blood would be what would give me power to do the unimaginable. Maybe it did; I learned to speak Spanish and French, paid my way through school on scholarships, and I do for a living that which I used to dream about. And, I make a mean paella and no one showed me how; that surely must be encoded in my genes, a gift from you.

Be well. I hope you went on to have a happy life.

Your unknown daughter,
Cassandra

HEALING EMOTIONAL WOUNDS FROM THE PAST

Remember, time doesn't heal all wounds. Love heals all wounds.

Do the following meditation and let it heal you even where you don't yet know healing needs to be done:

- Sit in Easy Pose and raise your right arm up to sixty degrees in front of you.
- Bring your left arm behind you in a sixty-degree angle pointed downward. The two arms should form a straight, sixty-degree line front and back. Keep your elbows straight and the index finder of each hand extended, with the thumb locking down the other fingers.
- Close your eyes and focus downward as if you are looking through the center of your chin. Breathe slowly and deeply. Do this for three minutes.
- Then, maintaining the same arm position, extend your pinkie finger on both hands with the index fingers. Eyes remain focused at the chin; do this for another three minutes.
- Finally, extend all your fingers and tighten the muscles of your body while you stretch out the arms towards Infinity for another three minutes. Inhale as deeply as you can, then exhale slowly and evenly; repeat this breath twice more, and you're finished! Again, start at one minute for each posture, if you like, and build up to three minutes.

Healing emotional wounds from the past

CREATING
A NEUTRAL
MIND

I remember the first thoughts that flashed through my head when I knew for sure I was pregnant: The first was, "Thank you dear God! This is a miracle! This is the happiest day of my whole life!" But it was followed by the little gremlins of worry, "How am I going to do this? I'm too old! I'm too nutty! We don't have enough money! Where will we live? I'm scared! I'm confused! I don't know anything! Will my baby be healthy?"

Even after I fell into the joy of carrying a baby, my husband and I still had stressed-out moments about one thing or another. We were moving out of an apartment when I found out I was pregnant, and we really had nowhere to go. We were on a very tight budget, and everything we could afford just seemed shabby, dank, and drab. With the baby coming now, I would just not settle for a place with no sunlight and ugly carpeting. So, I told my husband we would stay in a tent in my friends' backyard—in L.A.!—until we could find a cheerful little place.

He dragged his feet about it, but since he had lived in the Alaskan bush for eleven years, it wasn't so bad. So, live in a tent is what we did. Our friends let us use their bathroom and kitchen whenever we wanted, and it turned out to be quite lovely, actually. Our tent was under a lemon tree and I built a little altar where we meditated and read. We continued to look for a place, and I trusted from the bottom of my heart that God would give us a little home.

And that's what He did—we called it the "bird's nest," because it was so snug. By the end of my ninth month, I could barely get in and out of the bathroom, let alone fit in front of the sink, but it was home, and that was where I gave birth to Wahe Guru Kaur, which means "the princess in the ecstasy of God's name." Your babies bring gifts with them—houses, jobs, opportunities, things you never even imagined!

When you think about it, stress is really the opposite of trust. "God doesn't give us more than we can handle," is an old expression. The only reason life becomes unmanageable is because we think we are the great Doer of all things, that we are in total control. Wrong. We have a great expression, "If you can't see God in all, you can't see God at all."

Take a moment to see the reality of the situation. If you have to, make a list of all the things you do have and all the resources that are available to you. Yogis use the word *maya* to describe the fantasy and delusion we buy into as a part of everyday life. Look, the ground is still beneath your feet, the sky is still in the heavens above. The world will in fact continue spinning. Live one breath at a time, and solutions will present themselves.

When you are confused, stop and press your Third Eye point on your forehead between your eyebrows with your thumb and shut your eyes, inhaling "Sat" and exhaling "Nam" for three minutes. It will remind you to come back to center. Ask for help from the Universe. We weren't meant to do everything alone. Sit in the middle of the confusion. I promise you, the answer will come.

Which reminds me, it is not selfish to get massages during your pregnancy, to take baths, to pamper yourself. It's a necessity. When you get a massage, for instance, it's good for your baby because it gets the blood circulating and relaxes sore or tight muscles. Foot massages are particularly divine, and anybody can figure out how to rub feet—just hand him some cream! And make sure you put your feet up in his lap. So, if people say they want to do something for you, here's their chance! Say, "Thank you, how about a massage?"

Everything you do for yourself you are doing for the soul within you, to relax, to eat well, to walk, to meditate, to be with good friends, to read wonderful books. Your baby is taking all of it in like a sponge.

MEDITATION FOR MENTAL BALANCE

As yoginis we learn to create a neutral mind. Every negative thought is met with a positive thought. For instance, standing by a fireplace you might think, "The flames could burn me," then in the next breath, "Look at how beautiful the fire is and the warmth it offers." While laboring a voice might say, "I can't do this, it's too hard," then you must follow with, "Yes, I can. Yes, I am stronger than I have ever been in my whole life." That is the teeter-totter of the positive and negative mind. It is the nature of the mind to have a thousand thoughts pass by in the blink of an eye. Our minds, like tuning a radio, pick up the strongest frequencies of where we are at the time. Meditation takes us back to the neutral mind, the balance point on that teeter-totter, which is the mind we will birth from, and the mind we must operate from as mothers.

- Sit quietly in Easy Pose.
- Extend your arms out to your sides like great wings, palms flat and facing the floor.
- Begin flapping just your wrists and hands rapidly, as though you were flying furiously through the air. Your arms will move slightly from the shoulders, but the action is in the wrists.
- Breathe in long, deep inhales and exhales and continue for three minutes.

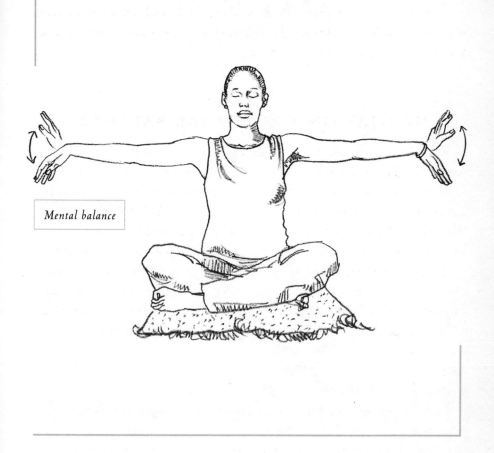

Mental balance

CULTIVATING
PATIENCE

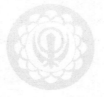

"The fertility of this
solid earth,
And the rain of that
blue immensity,
These two interact for
the benefit of
all things. . . ."

— MILAREPA

How often do you feel the dirt between your hands? See a sunset? Many of us are so detached from nature now. Fewer and fewer of us can say that on any given day we touch the Earth. We have given ourselves over to our asphalt and concrete reality and lost the origin of the human experience.

Before you have this baby, do one thing if you don't have any plants in your home: Get a plant. Any kind of plant will do as long as it's a real one with roots and stems and leaves, not one of those fake silk things. This is your practice in nurturing and connecting to the physical world. It is also a wonderful metaphor for your pregnancy. You find out how much sun it needs, what food makes it grow, how much water it requires to flourish. Watch your plant grow as you watch yourself grow. If you are already a gardener, good for you! Keep going.

Creation is a gift, but we still have to do the work of it. When a farmer goes to his fields, he can sow the seeds and then just hope that they grow, or he can water them, weed them, make sure the soil is supported to nurture the growth of the crop, and then pray over his fields. He gives great attention to the growing process. So it is with the baby inside you.

Plants teach us patience. That is our "dis-ease" in America: We have little patience with our children, our partners, our parents, even with the remote control (that's me, if I can't figure out how to make it work, I get mad and say in exasperation, "This stupid thing!"). We often get upset at the restaurant if the food doesn't come fast enough, or if there is traffic on the street. We are a nation built on impatience, on an "I want it yesterday" approach. When I go to India and take students who have never been there, I can see the frustration on many of their faces, "Why are people sitting around doing nothing? This country is so poor, why are they just sitting there?" It frustrates Westerners. Well, they are sitting because they are *enjoying* life. In the many trips I take to India, I love how time stands still there. The rush of "how much can I get done and how quickly" subsides. The mind winds down. Osho, a twentieth-century prophet, said what took six weeks to do two hundred years ago now takes one day. We have no space left in our minds. Try it on as a concept: Imagine not having to fill every single second of your time and just see what develops.

Often when we go into labor, our heads are not set to have a baby. That's why these nine months are so important. We can learn to do things that literally slow us down. We have one saying that my teacher gave us more than thirty-two years ago when he came to America, "Patience pays." That means I trust in the Creator and the timing that is much bigger than "I want it now."

The lesson of patience is one of the first a student on a spiritual path learns. When my teacher was a boy, he went to ask a wise old yogi some questions. The old yogi pointed to a tree and told him, "Wait up there until I return, and then I will answer your questions." The story goes that Yogi Bhajan waited in the tree for three days until the old man returned! The patience you will acquire as a mother . . . you cannot imagine now the length of it.

Start now with your plants. Tend to them. Watch them flourish in their own time. If for some reason your little lives in pots run up against some challenges and you don't know what to do, call upon an experienced gardener for some tips!

MEDITATION FOR BEING PATIENT

This Jupiter meditation will help bring your nervous system into balance and help you grow patience! Sitting in Easy Pose, eyes closed and rolled upward, extend your arms straight out to your sides, parallel to the ground, palms up, elbows straight. Using a powerful breath, begin to move only your Saturn finger, the middle finger. Inhale and you raise the middle finger and exhale as you lower it, coordinating the movement with the breath for seven minutes. Start with three minutes, if you like. You simply must do it to see how well it works in just three minutes.

Being patient

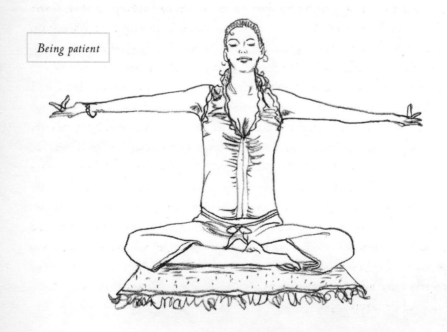

APPRECIATING
YOUR
PARTNER

Right about now, your husband or partner might be freaking out. While you are thinking about what to eat or feeling your baby moving for the first time, he is wrestling with issues he might never have considered before—Will he be able to provide for you and the baby? What's expected of him? Will he be a good father? Does he even have a clue what it is to be a father? Will he be like his own father, and if he doesn't want to be, how can he not be? And, perhaps biggest of all, how will the baby change you and your relationship to him? He can go through a range of feelings as he adjusts to his wife becoming a mother. Combining the sexual feelings he has for you as a lover with the idea that you will be a mother can sometimes take some rearranging in his own mind.

It was hard not to get irritated at my husband sometimes, because I remember being so full of my own experience of pregnancy, it didn't occur to me to think he might not be on the same wavelength at the same time. In the first trimester I was impossible. I cried a lot and was disappointed when he didn't get why I was crying—but then, even I didn't get why I was crying! By the fifth month, my emotions had stabilized and I was very happy.

Then Thanksgiving came, and it was unexpectedly a tough time for me. My past hit me like the proverbial ton of bricks. Thanksgiving morning I was preparing a sweet potato dish to take to our community feast. As I let it cool, I went into the bedroom to change my clothes, sat down on the bed, and I stared out the window. It was raining softly, one of the first rains of that year. Since I was raised in the Midwest where rain is plentiful, I miss it in the long L.A. summers absent of rain. I wanted to start dancing in the street, getting soaking wet, yelling "Yeah!" All of a sudden I began crying, just crying, and memories began their slow dance in front of my mind's eye: remembering the birth and death of my son; remembering a time years before when my brother was a teenager and had stolen a car. My parents had to drive to Nebraska to get him, so that when I came home from my first semester in college, I was greeted only by an empty house and a note on the kitchen table. But I was also crying for the rain itself, for the wet leaves, for the miracle inside of me, for all my happiness. It seemed I was crying for anything and everything for which there was to cry.

My husband found me sitting there wet from all my tears, and he was so divine. He listened to me, and he understood. He took the sweet potato dish to the feast and represented us both while I just lay in bed, feeling so good, so cleansed, so grateful. Tell your husbands they can always say, "My wife is pregnant and not able to come tonight." No more is needed. Most everyone accepts that easily. For me that was a day of cleansing and healing, and I felt so much better from then on.

The reality of relationships is exactly the opposite of what we have been taught about the knight on the white horse coming and sweeping us away. Think of yourself as having your own horse, able to swing by to pick him up if he falls off his. No man I have ever met is ready-made. Where their mother left off is where you pick up. Some of us have unions in which we have settled our differences through lifetimes of union and reunion, and this time around is a gift. For most of us in a relationship, it is work to stay together. Not just to coexist, but to grow together, to build something great together, to reveal the truth of our hearts to each other. It is worth the work and every ounce of commitment.

HAPPY COUPLE MEDITATION

Venus *kriyas* are partner meditations. If he doesn't already know, teach him the basics of sitting in Easy Pose, then come sitting back to back, making sure the base of your spines are together. If you are a single parent, do this with a close friend.

- Deeply inhale and exhale, then begin in unison to chant, "Sa-Ta-Na-Ma," for eleven minutes.
- Begin by chanting out loud for several minutes, then do it quietly in a whisper, then silently to yourselves, and finally returning to chant out loud to finish.

Happy couple meditation

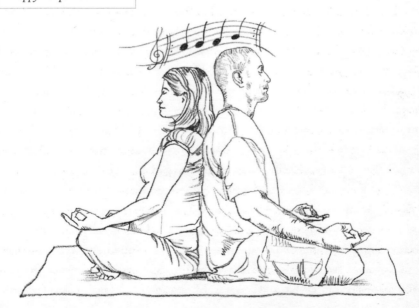

CREATING A POSITIVE PICTURE OF PREGNANCY AND BIRTH

TV might be the worst development for childbirth since midwives started to be burned at the stake. You think I'm kidding? I'm not. Think of scenes from the show *ER*, with a woman screaming and sweating, doctors running around everywhere—Will she make it? Will the baby make it? There's blood running like water. Oh, please. Unfortunately, normal birth doesn't make an exciting sixty-minute episode the way a rare birth complication does, or a character dying in childbirth, or getting stuck in a freeway traffic jam and delivering in a car!

The message that underlies all these TV images comes at us like a slow-acting poison we women ingest without realizing it. The toxic message is that in pregnancy and birth we are weakened creatures at the mercy of a bloody, scary traumatic event. So few of us have any previous experience to act as an antidote to these toxic messages. For most American women, the birth experience has been removed from the home for several generations and been turned into an institutionalized experience. A first-time mother rarely has any direct experience of childbirth to be able to say when she sees TV, "That's not how it is."

Some of the stories you might hear from people aren't likely to help any, either. Women love to share their birth stories, because birth is a transcendent time; something big and suspenseful does happen, guaranteed. However, some of us like to relate our labor story in an exaggerated way, "sixty hours to birth my child!" If you hear this kind of story, always ask, "How long was your *active* labor?" Active labor is where we have to breathe with our complete attention through every contraction. I have never met anyone who had sixty hours of active labor. Other women will tell you that they didn't feel anything at all and the baby popped right out. The reality is usually somewhere in between.

In our collective human history, a pregnant woman was considered anything but weak. In tribal times, birth was a period of honor for women. A woman in childbirth was given as much respect as a man in battle. Among the Aztecs, in fact, women in childbirth were given the same recognition as warriors who had returned from battle.

Start to cleanse your mind of the *ER* images. Talk to other women with positive and not exaggerated birth stories, read good books like author Anita Diamant's novel *The Red Tent* and *Spiritual Midwifery* by Inna May Gaskin to learn of our childbirth history as females, past and present. Let us begin to share in each other's lives, rediscovering our own knowledge and intuition.

BANISHING FEAR

- Sit in Easy Pose, with your eyes closed and rolled upward, and extend your arms out to the side, parallel to the ground.
- Close your hands, bringing the fingertips only to the base of your palm, thumbs up.
- Keep your spine straight and your chin slightly tucked.

- Inhale and bring your thumbs to your shoulders, returning your hands to the original position with an exhale.
- Go as fast as you can and don't let your thumbs touch your shoulders.
- Continue with powerful breathing for two minutes to stimulate your pituitary gland. Work up to seven minutes.

Banishing fear

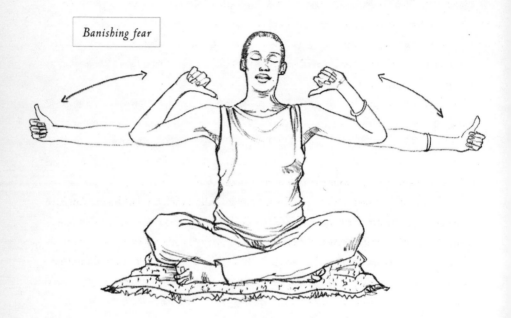

CONSIDERATIONS FOR HOW AND WHERE TO BIRTH

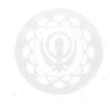

When you own your birth, you own your life.

It's not too early to begin considering how you will birth. You have choices for places to have your baby. If you start weighing your options now, you won't be in a last-minute rush. You'll be confident of the choice you made when the time comes, whether you decide to birth at home, in a hospital, or at a birthing center. The important step at first is just to realize you have options. We're very fortunate in the West to have the best of all worlds available to us, if we choose.

I never advocate a home birth, but I do encourage healthy women to look into it—and that just happens to be the majority of us. We have to understand that there is a difference between a normal birth and a typical birth; about 95 percent of births are without complications and can be done at home. In the United States, home or birthing center deliveries with midwives are only 7 percent of births. That doesn't mean home births are unusual in any regard. In northern European countries, for example, about 70 percent of births take place at home with midwives.

I was fascinated to learn the vast number of folk remedies used in ancient

Roman times that were written down. Much of it was totally revolting: A drink made with sow's dung was supposed to relieve pain during labor, as was sow's milk mixed with honey wine, and most revolting of all, "the liquid that flows from a weasel's genitals." Imagine! A vulture's feather was put under the foot of a laboring woman, and the sloughed skin from a snake was tied around her thigh. Despite the fact that the "remedies" were a sanitation nightmare and probably didn't do much good—apart from the fact that people believed they worked, so they had a powerful placebo effect—the maternity care still had some things going for it: The ancient texts describe it as being personal and attentive to the woman laboring. She was at a home, a place where she was comfortable, and she was surrounded by female relatives and midwives who supported and encouraged her. That emotionally supportive, personal, secure atmosphere did more for her than anything. Ironically, despite the long way we've come from sow's dung, that warm, individualized, personal care is what is so often missing in our modern approach to childbearing.

If you want to investigate a home birth, make sure you take your husband or your partner with you to talk to a midwife rather than try to convince him of it after the fact—otherwise it will sound like myth, like magic, hearsay. Unless he too understands the process, he might think you have lost your mind.

In any case, you need to ask questions of the facility where you will birth, and of the doctor or midwife who will catch your baby. If health professionals become defensive when questioned, do not have the time to answer you, or if you do not agree with what you are told, ask yourself: Do I want to put myself in this person's care? Make sure you ask your questions gracefully and skillfully to avoid putting anyone on the defensive with a harsh tone.

Some questions to consider asking are:

- Will you welcome my labor assistant in the birthing room?
- Are eating, drinking, and walking encouraged during labor if I choose?
- Do you require an IV hook-up as soon as I arrive?
- What is the circumstance under which an IV will be needed?
- What are your views on Pitocin and epidurals?

- What's your caesarean rate?
- How do you define "overdue"?
- How long do you let a woman be overdue before you advocate interventions?
- Who covers for you if you go on vacation or need to be away during my due date, and are you close enough to your substitute to know if they share your views on childbirth?
- Can I give birth in a squatting or vertical position if I want to?
- How do you define a "slow" labor and do you set time limits before you suggest inducing?
- Under what conditions would the baby's father and I be separated from the baby?
- What do you do if my water breaks at home?

Above all, trust your intuition. The ancient teachings say that a woman can sense something "sixteen moons before it will happen," a metaphorical way of saying we have finely tuned instincts that make us much more intuitive than men. After all is said and done, what is your gut reaction to the hospital? To the doctor? To the midwife or birthing center?

Wherever you choose to birth, make it work within that context. Don't try to have a home birth in the hospital, and vice versa; don't expect your home to have the high-tech of a hospital. If you have chosen a hospital, some place in your mind tells you there is a reason you have chosen it. The important thing is not to be rigid. Investigate all your options, mentally project the birth you want to have, but then allow your mind to expand and accommodate all possibilities.

Always remember that children are born exactly the way they need to be born. We are born into this lifetime to grow, and it is only through experience that we grow. Once labor starts, the process is bigger than any one person's plan. Sometimes, a soul coming through needs a certain experience for its journey, or maybe the mother needs it for hers, or the father needs it for his. We call it a complication, but it is a thread among the many thousands of threads that create the rich tapestry of a life.

MEDITATION FOR MAKING DECISIONS

This meditation will help build your inner knowingness:

- Sit in Easy Pose with your eyes closed focusing at the Third Eye point.
- Bring your hands into prayer pose at the center of your chest and then slide the left hand up until the entire palm is higher than the right. Your right palm will be touching your left palm just below the wrist.
- Inhale "Sat," and exhale "Nam."
- Breathe as long and slowly as you can for three minutes.

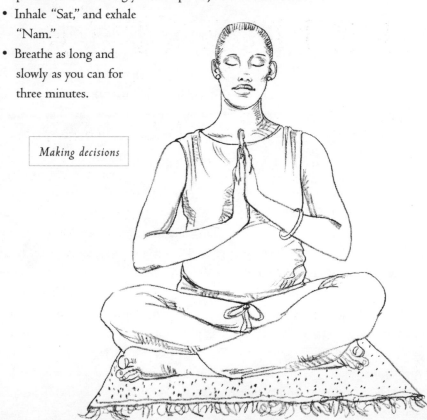

Making decisions

THE
SECOND
TRIMESTER

*Believe that you
are the miracle,
just because
you are a woman.*

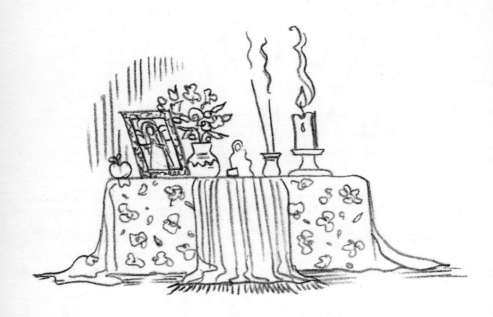

A SOUL
ARRIVES

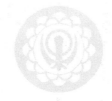

I n this very ancient tradition in which I live, we have a special celebration during pregnancy to honor the soul who arrives on the one hundred and twentieth day after conception, which corresponds to the fourth month of pregnancy, about a month into your second trimester. Before the end of the first trimester, the fetus that supports the soul hasn't been completely fortified, and this is when the majority of miscarriages happen. Before that date, the entering soul is still unaffected by worldly influences, existing only in radiance.

When the soul enters the body, a baby's subconscious mind begins to develop and absorb a multitude of messages, the way a dry sponge soaks up water. Usually morning sickness has subsided, and we are getting our bearings on life; the waters become more calm.

In our homes, the father of the arriving soul, friends, and family of the mother organize the celebration so we don't have to do anything. They prepare delicious food, arrange flowers, and light candles. They call together members of the community, who bring gifts to honor the mother. Singing, poems, and scriptures can be read—whatever they feel the new mother would love—along with plenty of good food served. Everyone prays for her physical, mental, and spiritual well-being so she is strong and able to pass those qualities through herself to the baby.

It is one of our most beautiful celebrations, and one I encourage you to take on in whatever context is appropriate for your life and your beliefs. One of our students, Fabienne, did exactly that. Here is her experience, in her own words:

"The first three months of pregnancy were, for me, very medicalized. There were tests after tests after tests. I was awash in the technology of childbirth. So, at the one hundred and twentieth day, we decided to have a party. It was to herald a new time when I could just surrender to the experience of pregnancy and enjoy it. It was about moving out of the medical and into the celebration of creation.

"I found it so empowering. I dressed in a beautiful orange gown from Tibet, there was fresh food and flowers everywhere, and I sat on a 'throne'—okay, an ottoman—surrounded by pillows and incense. A friend played the harmonium, an Indian keyboard instrument, and sang songs. I could really feel a shift from my focus being centered on what could be wrong with my pregnancy into appreciating and experiencing the power of creation.

"We kept the guest list very small. We kept the group to only those friends and family members who could embrace what we were doing and who were nonjudgmental about the process. We didn't want to feel guarded or uncomfortable, and we certainly didn't want anyone else to feel that way, either.

"We asked our guests not to buy gifts—although they did—but just bring good intentions for the baby. We ate and laughed and talked, and then we did the Adi Shakti meditation, a lovely yogic prayer to the female energy that creates the world, for thirty-one minutes, which represents a yogic time of completion. It left us all feeling an inward focus, and put us in a place of welcoming the soul.

"I think it was great for my husband. It was the first time he felt like he could participate in some meaningful way in the process. He even wrote a song called 'Welcome to this World' for the baby, which he now plays every day. The chorus goes:

Welcome to this world
Whether you're ready or not
Welcome to this world
Come give it all that you got
Welcome to this world
Before you know it you'll be
singing right back to me
Welcome to this world

"I think our son will come out singing the words! The melody is so innocently sweet I don't think there was a dry eye left in the room. I think also that it helped him with the transition of seeing me as his wife to mother of his child.

"Gurmukh called that night and talked with my husband. She 'ordered' me to completely rest the next day, and put him in charge of seeing to it that would happen. She said so much energy was going into the baby right now I did not need to do more, to just sit and watch the rose unfold.

"So the next day, I took off work and spent the whole day lounging around in bed. I took a bath, and then I had a great dinner with my husband. It was the first time I felt like I was pregnant. It was the first time for us to focus not on all the things that could go wrong, but on all the things that had gone right. Not only with the pregnancy, but with our lives. The impact of it still lingers."

CONNECTING WITH YOUR BABY

At this stage, you can connect mentally to your child. With your partner and a group of friends, enjoy this meditation to open the heart chakra, the center of compassion:

- Sit in Easy Pose.
- Press your palms together in front of your nose, arms out horizontal with

elbows parallel to the ground with the tips of your middle fingers level with your brow.

- Focus at your Third Eye point, eyes closed.
- Breathe deeply and evenly; start at three minutes and work up to eleven minutes.
- To end, stretch your body lightly and gently for two minutes, in whatever way feels comfortable.

Connecting with your baby

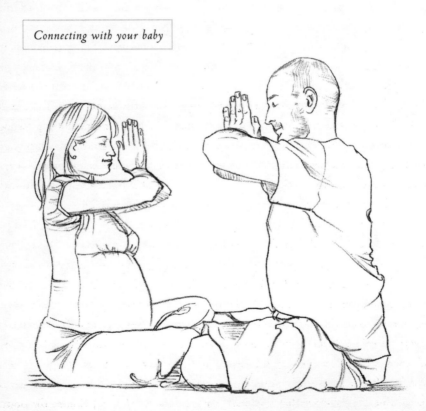

NOURISH
YOURSELF

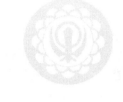

When I was a child, we had a lovely, big old elm tree in our yard. The trunk of the tree split in a fork going off into two directions, resembling strong arms reaching up to the sky. In the center of that fork, robins would build a nest in the spring after the snow melted and the day's sun lingered longer. When the eggs finally hatched and the chicks were born, the elm became the place they would fly from and be received into the world.

That nest and the life that sprang from it depended on the elm being healthy and able to shelter and protect the birds. Its roots took in moisture and nutrients from the soil, its branches raised up to the sun, and its green leaves soaked in the rays.

The well-being of the family, and of society itself, depends upon us as women becoming and remaining healthy, like the sheltering elm containing the life of the birds. So, nourish yourself. Women's bodies are different from men's in that the Earth's energy moves up through our bodies and inward. Our female energy is the "drawing in" energy, also called centripetal force. I've heard that the reason Navajo women wear big, heavy skirts is because doing so increases the body's access to this earth energy through the circle that the skirt creates on the Earth in relation to the body.

Centripetal energy is the grounding force that makes women the centers of their households. When a woman elevates her life for the better, her entire family benefits, because she sets a new level of awareness and clarity in the home.

Good nutrition is one of the central pillars of a healthy pregnancy. We know that having a baby puts new demands on your body—a lot more is going on. Fortunately, good nutrition isn't a complicated issue in this country.

First things first:

- Do your best to cut out junk food, white sugar, and fast food. We are a nation of faster is better—go more, have more, be more. And that extends to our food choices. You want a fast food? Have an apple, organic if possible—you can even eat the wrapper it comes in! Better to eat fruit than drink it as juice.
- Support your body with foods filled with *prana*, life energy, fresh and alive and organic when at all possible. Drink lots of pure water—even if you have to run to the bathroom every five minutes, make sure you keep drinking water.
- If you start swelling in your fingers and feet, look at what you are eating first. The culprit is very often iodized table salt. Even if you don't use the salt shaker, do you eat out? Do you eat prepared foods? Salt, salt, salt. It heightens flavor and is used more than we can imagine in sauces—in just about everything.
- Eat cucumbers and watermelon; they help with water retention.
- If you need to fly, remember that the air is dehydrating on a plane. Take a big zipper-lock bag of cucumber slices with you. During your naps, or at home in bed at night, or on a plane, also put them on your eyes for comfort and soothing—they fit perfectly!

Organic foods and foods that are not genetically altered are the best for you and your baby. Fresh fruits and vegetables are full of *prana*, life force, and when you eat these foods you receive that energy and goodness, just what you need to sustain you and baby. Fill your refrigerator with fresh, live food. When you open your refrigerator door, let your shelves be as colorful as a bouquet; it will feel like a blessing.

In most cases eating more vegetables than fruit is best. Wanting sweets to excess can be an indicator you're low on protein—60 grams a day in most cases will supply what your pregnant body needs. Protein powders, like Naturade brand in soy, can provide up to 25 grams when you whip it up in a fruit shake in the blender, and they are delicious. Mung beans and rice are the most tasty and easily digestible form of protein in the world. You can eat this combination every day to feel good and strong. Here's the recipe:

MUNG BEAN AND RICE MEAL

4½ quarts water
1 cup mung beans
2 cups basmati rice
½ cup chopped ginger root
1 to 2 onions, chopped
½ bulb garlic, chopped
2 to 8 cups vegetables
2 tablespoons ghee or oil
½ teaspoon crushed red chiles
2 teaspoons turmeric
1 tablespoon ground coriander
½ teaspoon black pepper
2 teaspoons curry powder
½ teaspoon ground cumin
2 teaspoons sea salt or more to taste

Set the water to boil in a 6- or 8-quart pot. Clean beans of any debris and rinse well. Add them to the water and boil until they start to split, about 30 minutes. Meanwhile, prepare the other ingredients. Clean rice in the same manner as the beans. Peel and chop the ginger root, onions, and garlic. Add rice to the beans. Chop the other ingredients in the order they are listed and add them to the mix. Heat the oil or ghee in a small pan over medium heat, add all the spices, and let them sizzle for 30 seconds, stirring. Add this to the bean mix. As the rice starts to break up, lower the heat to medium and stir occasionally. Continue to cook, uncovered, until all the ingredients are very well done and a bit mushy. Add sea salt or Bragg's Amino Acids to taste. Total preparation time is about 1½ hours, including stirring occasionally. You can also put it in a crockpot to cook overnight.

If you don't eat red meat or have been a vegetarian, don't stop now that you're pregnant. So many women go back to eating steak after years of not eating it, thinking it's the only way they can get enough protein. Veggie burgers, protein powders, beans and rice, almonds and other nuts, and broccoli all provide more digestible protein than meat!

Increasingly science tells us what the yogis have known for millennia: To a large extent, lifelong health is shaped in the womb. The risk of tooth decay and prostate cancer are just two of the diseases linked to life in utero. The Chinese for centuries have believed that not only health but character is formed in the womb. They know that certain food and herbs can affect our physical health and emotional well-being. Special *"chin"* tonics, for instance, are said to open the heart chakra so that love, kindness, gentleness, and compassion start to rule an individual. Dunwood *reishi* mushroom is the most coveted *chin* tonic by Chinese women during their pregnancy. *Reishi* regulates the immune system to ward off disease, but it's also said that *"reishi* babies," as they're called, are calmer, and healthier, and just seem to radiate a special charisma. For more information on Chinese herbals, read Ron Teegarden's book *Chinese Tonic Herbs.*

Some mothers approach eating during pregnancy from the standpoint that they don't want to gain too much weight. If you eat fresh, whole live food, as organic as possible, and lots of salads, rather than the processed stuff that lines most of the shelves in the grocery store, you won't put on unneeded weight. Make choices for your child's life. If you find that your weight gain is too large, try eating your main meal in the afternoon, and eat only fruit and vegetables at night. That is how our family eats and it has worked for years. Look closely at how much of your diet is made up of bread and dairy products, like hard cheese and butter, especially if you are experiencing constipation and/or hemorrhoids and heartburn. Soy products can be a good substitute for dairy.

This reminds me of Lila, a student who just two minutes into the first exercise at class was exhausted. "Lila," I said, "what's wrong?"

"Oh," she replied, "I haven't wanted to eat anything but marshmallows for the last two days, so that's all I've had." She started to cry. "Everybody says you should give in to your cravings while you're pregnant! I've just been on a marshmallow kick."

Maybe it didn't matter so much forty years ago what we ate, because there was not so much junk and chemical fillers in the food. The pace of life was much different than it is today, with our cell phones and Internet and faxes and beepers. I look at all the processed snacks people give their kids now, and I think, is it any wonder so many get diagnosed with Attention Deficit Disorder? Here's the equation: Kids + sugar + computers = insanity. It's very important to be aware of what you eat, because that's what feeds your baby. Earaches, bronchial infections, and asthma can all be common indicators of weakened immune systems. Establishing healthy habits while your baby is inside you helps create patterning for the rest of your life—and your baby's! What a child eats after he is born is very much what a mother chooses while she is pregnant and nursing.

You'll see, if you don't already know, that living with children is like living with spies in your house—your every behavior is being recorded somewhere! Kids will copy everything you do, guaranteed. Use this time for new food patterning for the rest of his life and for yours.

We have a beautiful student, a labor and delivery nurse, who was already the mother of two when she started coming to our Wednesday class for women. She came up to me after class to say she had decided to become a vegetarian, and her family had agreed to come along also. After almost a year, her family is blossoming—she looks radiant and reports that her family is calmer and healthier than ever before. She came back to class again, but this time for prenatal! "I'm happy to be doing it this time as a vegetarian," she reported. She recently delivered a beautiful child at home. Her friend, who is an OB, came over at the start of her labor, but they never made it to the hospital—it happened that quickly!

Find out what is in food. For instance, we have been taught to think of milk as such a wholesome food, but so much is in dairy products now—hormones, antibiotics given to cows, steroids, you name it. If you drink milk, make it organic. If you don't become an aware parent, you might end up with some surprises you don't like. You must take responsibility now. The good news is that when you do start eating better, Dad starts eating better, and so does the whole family. I was telling the dads in my pregnancy couples' workshop recently that they must even reconsider taking the kids to get a "Happy Meal." Think about this: McDonald's entices families to eat steroid-, hormone-, preservative-laden products, and then has a house for children with cancer. What's wrong with this picture?

I have been a vegetarian for thirty-five years, not eating any meat, fish, or eggs. At the age of fifty-four I became a vegan, which means I now also don't eat dairy products. You might ask yourself where I get my protein. Broccoli is just one example—it provides more digestible protein than meat. In my tradition, we don't eat anything that runs, swims, or flies away from us. As my daughter often says, "How can anyone eat something that has a mother and has eyes just like I do?" Our faith has raised three generations of vegetarian children now, and I am convinced we have some of the happiest and healthiest children in the world.

Your commitment to your children will keep you healthy and happy and holy. Wouldn't it be nice to live with greater health not just in pregnancy, but for all time? See what blessings children bring? An opportunity for great changes in your life!

TREE POSE:
EXERCISE FOR BALANCE,
STRENGTH, AND FOCUS

Become a tree and experience standing tall, majestic, and solid!

- Come standing with your weight evenly distributed along your feet, and your spine straight as if you are being pulled toward the ceiling on an invisible string. You can start out next to a wall for balance.
- Bring your hands in prayer pose to the center of your chest, then lift one foot up and place it on your opposite ankles, knee, or inner thigh, depending on your balance.
- Softly lower your eyes and focus out and down about five feet in front of you. As your balance steadies, lift your arms out and straight up to the sky, arms parallel and palms facing inward.
- Do this for two minutes on each side as you breathe long and deep. Inhale and exhale from your belly, your baby's home.

Tree pose

BELIEVE
IN MIRACLES

B elieve in a miracle. More than that, believe you *are* the miracle, just because you are a woman! To us in my tradition, "wo" means great beyond words, and "man" means mind or being. Put together, it means a woman's being is so great no words can describe it.

The amazing is all around us if we stop to listen. A woman in class was told she wouldn't be able to carry her baby to term because she had a cyst in her uterus. The mother refused to accept this diagnosis, which she called a death sentence for her baby. She started on a daily regime of yoga, walking, a forty-day meditation, prayer, and visualization of dissolving that cyst. She also ate a vegan diet high in plant proteins. On her next ultrasound, the doctor could find no evidence of the cyst. She carried to term and delivered a beautiful daughter.

Another student was told she would not be able to deliver vaginally because of her pelvic structure, but she was set on having a natural birth. She began hiking like a wild woman, up hills and down, and every time I looked at the faces in my yoga class, hers was among them. She meditated, prayed, and ate live, whole foods. When it came time to labor, the baby was in a fine position and came through the birth canal without incident. I am not promising if you practice yoga and learn to meditate you are guaranteed protection from all challenges in life, but I am telling you, as Shakespeare once wrote, that "There are more things in Heaven and Earth than has been dreamt of in our philosophies."

A rock star I used to teach told me a story about being in her tour bus while her band was on the road in Canada. One night, they passed an accident on the highway, and she was the only one who was awake. "Stop the bus!" she told the driver, and she ran out to where a car was overturned. This skinny little rock 'n' roller actually saved three people's lives by lifting the car they were pinned under so that they could be pulled out. The next day, of course, this same woman couldn't even lift a fender. You have to ask, Who or what was that person inside her that came forward to lift up that car? We all have that infinitely strong identity inside us. It is the Infinite, limitless, all-powerful that comes in these emergency moments, arriving before the thought, "No, not possible." Since there is no time for the mind to enter the experience, we act without that thought. If she had stopped long enough to say, "Wait, what am I doing? I can't do this, it's too hard," she wouldn't have been able.

Each of us has the ability to go right to the source, passing right by the thought. If you get caught in the thought, you will think, "This hurts too much," "I can't do it," "I'm tired," and a million other things. Not too long ago a man fainted in class because of the subject I was discussing. I was describing the process used nowadays to slaughter animals for meat, from the book *Diet for a New America*. I don't go on and on about being a vegetarian. Still, I do know some things that are important to consider about our food choices. The graphic description of the slaughterhouse was so visual, he fainted. I just jumped off my teacher's bench as soon as I saw him waver, went right over to him, and helped bring him back to consciousness. Now if I had thought, "I don't know what to do, I'm not a doctor," I wouldn't have been able to help at all. That will be your challenge: to be the person you are before getting stopped by thoughts that tell you what you aren't.

In this country, we have the boon of too much information. We go to the doctor who makes one small comment, like, "Gee, the baby seems really big," and all of a sudden, we're in a panic. "Your amniotic fluid level seems low." Panic. "You might have difficulty in labor, given the angle of your pelvis." Panic. "This baby could be breech." Panic. Sometimes issues are genuine. Many times in the course of events, they turn out not to be serious issues at all, or are temporary and pass. Though the medical society we live in can seem to make pregnancy and birthing a technical experience, it is not. The marvel of this experience is that this being who is so close to us cannot be seen. We don't have a window in, or a pouch like a kangaroo. When you can't see and touch, you have the opportunity to connect deeply on another level. We are so used to looking in mirrors, but you will never know what is going inside if you keep looking out. You have to birth from within. Yoga and meditation can be the golden chain that links the two of you together in this profound miracle we call creation.

MEDITATION FOR BEING HAPPY

This is called the Smiling Buddha *kriya*. The story goes that a brahman found Siddhartha nearly starved and in an unhappy way, unable to walk after a forty-day fast. The brahman nursed him back to health, and when Siddhartha finally began to smile again, the brahman taught him this *kriya*. Siddhartha went on to become Buddha who found Enlightenment under the bodhi tree!

- Sit in Easy Pose and curl the ring and pinkie fingers in, pressing them down with your thumb while keeping your first two fingers straight.
- Bring your arms up so that your elbows are pushed back and a thirty-degree angle is made between the upper arm and forearm, keeping the forearms parallel to each other. Palms face forward.
- Close your eyes and concentrate on the Third Eye point very powerfully.
- Chant mentally, "Sa-Ta-Na-Ma." The sound "Sa" expresses the infinite;

"Ta" expresses life; "Na" expresses diminishing; "Ma" expresses light and regeneration.

- Do this for eleven minutes, then inhale deeply, exhale, open and close your fists a few times, and then relax. You will be smiling!

Being happy

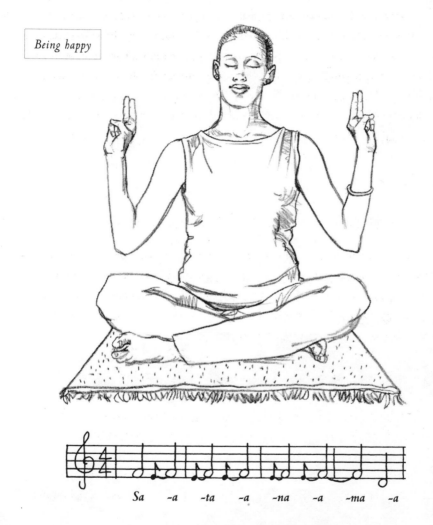

Sa   -a   -ta   -a   -na   -a   -ma   -a

REVEL
IN THE JOY

*"What a child learns
in the womb
cannot be learned
on earth."*

—YOGI BHAJAN

Candace comes to class eight months pregnant wearing a little stretchy pink top with her bare belly painted with henna designs, as if it were a supernova exploding in space. She wears beaded bangles on her wrists that clink when she moves, and when the music comes on and we dance, she shimmies and laughs and laughs. Would that every one of us could let go and be as free as she is! Candace is ecstasy personified.

Who told us pregnancy has to be so serious? The pace of your mind's thoughts matches the physical rhythm of your life. Create a space that is slower, more joyous. Dancing and bouncing and laughing are good for your lymphatic system, and your baby needs to be bounced, massaged, and caressed for all the reasons you do, and to stimulate brain development. This is true whether they are in or out of the womb. Babies love to dance, in or out of you.

Now is your time to celebrate your pregnancy. Wear whatever you want to, whatever you feel beautiful in—because you *are* beautiful. So often we get stuck in a rut of wearing black because it's sophisticated or slimming, or the same style day after day. Honor your body and stimulate your health by using the power of color now: Yogis have known forever that each of the eight chakras, or energy centers, in the body is represented by a corresponding color, and that color helps to activate the energy. Here's a brief summary to help get you started:

- The first chakra is called the root chakra. Located at the base of the tailbone, it represents life energy, sexuality, and strength. Red is its color.
- The second chakra is associated with ovulation, and is located at your uterus, where your baby lives. Orange is its color.
- The third chakra is found at the solar plexus, and represents emotions. Yellow is its color.
- The fourth chakra is the heart center, and has the power of healing and prosperity. Green is its color.
- The fifth chakra is that of communication and the power to speak truth, found at the throat. Blue is its color.
- The sixth chakra is the Third Eye point, and is the power of hidden knowledge and intuition, our meditative mind. Indigo is its color.
- The seventh chakra is found at the crown of the head and represents spirituality, the God consciousness within us. Violet is its color.
- The eighth chakra is your protective shield, the magnetic field produced by each living being. White is its color, representing the union of all colors in the spectrum.

What color do you *feel* like wearing? Is there something that draws you to green today? Violet? Orange, perhaps, even though you never thought you'd wear *that* color? Maybe it's your baby telling you something. . . . Trust yourself, and go for it!

A poem I often read in class says, "Banish the word struggle from your vocabulary. All that you do now must be done in a sacred manner and celebration. You are the one you have been waiting for."

One important part of getting to know your body is to feel your sensuality, feel the power to grow a baby, and feel the power you possess to bring her out into your arms. It is grace in action. The more we feel the glory and the magic of being a woman, the more we will come to know ourselves. You can even stop in the middle of a mall and do tree pose if you want! The more all that glory is felt and experienced on the inside, the more fear goes away.

When you live in joy, you are imparting that to your child. Children learn your real values by feeling them, without a word being spoken.

Choose carefully what words you speak now since the baby is listening to your vibrations. It's best not to read horror novels or books or magazines that are like junk food for the mind. Say to yourself, "Would I read this to my child?" Perhaps read something you have written that you've never read to anyone before. Get some old-fashioned story books. Poetry. Classic literature. Spiritually uplifting books. Reread some of your favorite books. Read them out loud if you like. This will help later when you tell bedtime stories—you'll have some memorized! What's better, your children will already know them.

Carefully pick the television shows and movies you watch, too—funny, romantic, and happy. Nothing violent! People think I'm joking when I tell them to take a pillow to put over your belly so you can muffle the sound so your baby doesn't hear it—especially during the previews because they always turn the sound up so loud. All those sounds go right through your belly and the baby's ears hear it. If you think I'm exaggerating about the importance of this, take a look at *The Message from Water*, a book published in Japan by writer Masauro Emoto. Emoto photographed water crystals as different music was played, as they were prayed over, and as they were spoken to. When words like "I love you" were spoken or beautiful music was played, the lovely, snowflake-like crystals formed, but when the water was exposed to heavy metal music and hateful words, they broke into jagged, ugly fragments. What does that mean for our bodies that are composed of 70 percent water? Think about it. What you do now, you do in the name of your baby.

DANCE OF JOY

The stretching and twisting and rocking you yourself did when you were in the womb are exactly the postures and exercises that sustain your body for a long, healthy, flexible life. So do what your baby is doing—move however it feels good to move. Don't let a day go by without dancing! Put on some music and dance and dance. Play whatever music you like. Be your own DJ. Let the music be uplifting and the rhythm strong but sweet, or primal, or ethnic, something that brings the joy out of you. I love the Beatles. Keep going for eleven minutes or more and move your hips. Don't let even one part of your body go unmoved!

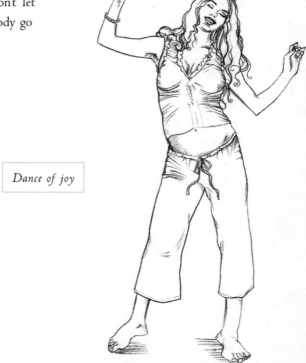

Dance of joy

YOUR MOST
IMPORTANT
JOB

*"How beautiful
it is to do nothing,
and then rest
afterward."*

—SPANISH PROVERB

I ask the class, How many of you are feeling:

Beautiful?
Fat?
Happy?
Tired?
Sensual?
Sick?
Sexy?
Energized?

Many of the hands go up when I say "fat," because our only point of reference, especially if this is the first baby, is that we are getting fat. But you are not getting fat, you are growing big in an incredibly *right* way.

The first trimester is a challenge, because it is an adjustment of self: "I" was one and now suddenly "I" am two. The second trimester is what I call the "Popple" time. When my daughter was small, there was a doll called a Popple, a big ball of furriness. If you rolled a flap of the ball back, pop! A fuzzy bear would unfold and the flap would be its bonnet. When women start to show, we say she did a "Popple," because it happens literally overnight. One morning you wake up and look in the mirror and you realize the whole world will know from this day forth that you are pregnant. The last trimester presents a challenge just because the baby is so big and you are so ready to have him, or her—or them—in your arms. In the second trimester, the challenge is watching your body grow and respecting that growth as important work.

Right now the job of growing your baby within your healthy body is of utmost importance, more important than any career consideration. This isn't old-fashioned; I am not suggesting your career isn't important. I am saying to consider honoring your motherhood as a role that is the most central and necessary in our human society. You decided to have a child, now give it your primary focus for these nine months of your life.

Pregnancy doesn't last forever. It's only nine months out of our lives. This is especially true for your first child. After that, your attention will also be given to your children on the outside of you. Still, see if you can find time each day for yourself and the "inside" child.

It is said that duty performed is God lived. Caring for your pregnant body is a spiritual experience if only you let it be one. While I carried Wa, I would sit and do a long *sadhana* meditation each morning at home before the sun came up. That became the priority in my life.

Sometimes we like to see how much we can do while we are pregnant, as if to say, "I am pregnant but am just like I was before. I won't miss a beat. I am Wonder Woman!" Maybe it is fear that we will lose the equality in society that has been won through so much struggle, or fear we will lose momentum along our professional path, or status. I appreciate all these considerations, but let us not devalue the miracle of motherhood in the process. Some of us fear a loss of intimacy with our partners and that their eyes will wander to others. If we lived in our true natures as women we would never have that fear, because a woman's nature would never betray her sister, even if she didn't know her personally. We must return to our root essence to heal this world and bring in a whole new kind of human being. Learn to be more, not do more.

No matter what sort of work you do, it is ideal if you can stop a few months before you have the baby so that your sole occupation is the baby. That isn't always possible. But can you slow down, work fewer hours, take naps or put your feet up at work? You'll be surprised at how much your value system changes after your little one arrives. The view from motherhood is so much bigger, and more far reaching, than what we see before our child comes to us. You will never regret the moments you take now, affirms Julie, who first came to prenatal classes fourteen years ago during her pregnancy with her son. "Slowing down gave me the luxury of connection. It gave me the time and the space to really tune in to my child," she says. "When you are pregnant, it's a balancing act between strengthening yourself and nurturing yourself. You have to work at your physical and emotional strength—but you also have to wrap yourself in soft cotton wool!"

MEDITATION FOR BEING ENOUGH JUST AS YOU ARE

- Sit in Easy Pose and relax your right arm on your right knee.
- Take your left hand and have it face your heart center about six inches from your chest.
- As you say "I am," move your hand toward your chest until it is only four inches from your heart.
- On a second "I am," take the hand twelve inches out from the chest. Inhale and draw the hand to the original position. With each movement of your hand you are extending yourself beyond all the limits you have set for your body.

- Continue this cycle for eleven minutes, starting at five if you like.
- As you do this, imagine that when your hand is close to your heart it is representing the "little me." When your hand is furthest away from you, it represents the big, ever-expanding nonlimited Self. In this meditation it's as if the "little me," the finite, limited self, merges to become one with the "big me," the infinite Self, over and over again. You will have an experience of how great, strong, and vast you really are.

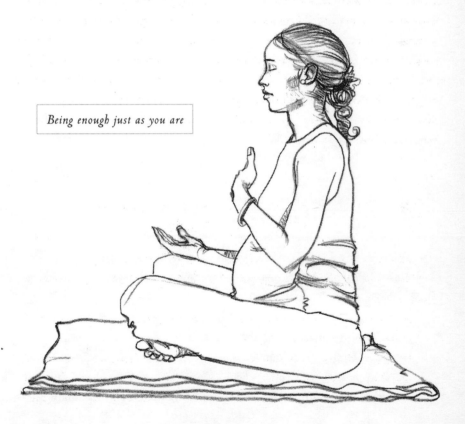

Being enough just as you are

SQUATTING
FOR
STRENGTH

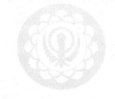

In the Victorian times, the only ladylike way to deliver a baby was thought to be from a supine position, flat on your back. But since the beginning of time, women have squatted to birth. Tribal childbirths, as any anthropologist can tell you, almost always occur in a special kind of birthing stool, kneeling, or squatting. I don't think it's a coincidence their labors tend to be much, much shorter than ours. Delivery can take place in a few minutes with the mother squatting, researcher Judith Goldsmith writes in *Childbirth Wisdom from the World's Oldest Societies*.

Whether or not you are able to actually give birth in a squatting position doesn't really matter. What matters is practicing this movement throughout your pregnancy because of the strength squatting gives you. There are many advantages to doing this:

- There is no compression on the vena cava and the aorta, the major blood supply system that runs through the center of your body.
- Squatting mobilizes the entire pelvic region, widening it as much as 25 percent.
- During labor, squatting produces minimum muscle strain, maximum pres-

sure inside the pelvis, and creates a perfect angle of descent for the baby. It makes gravity work for you, not against you.

• Squatting gives the baby optimal oxygen throughout the process and also relaxes the perineum area to lessen the potential for tearing.

Though squatting may not be the position your body tells you to go into during labor, the practice of squatting is very important—unless you are on bed rest or your baby is breech in the last six weeks of your pregnancy. Squatting tells your baby that the position is perfect, but squatting when your baby is breech gives an incorrect message to your baby and will perhaps set the breech even more if it is done in the last six weeks. Not only does squatting strengthen and lessen stiffness in your legs, but it also helps tone and stretch your back muscles and hips. Squatting takes pressure off your spinal discs, which can help ease your aching back, and helps elimination amazingly. I encourage each mother to do fifteen squats daily, because they align the pelvis, strengthen legs, and simply condition all muscles involved in the birth process. In other words, squats can only make you healthier and stronger.

Don't be surprised if this is difficult for you at first. Americans have lost the primal art of squatting, because we sit in chairs all the time, putting the back in a weak position and sapping our spines of their innate energy. The natural curve at the base of the spine is flattened, and knees at ninety-degree angles cut off the circulation to the legs below. All of American health would be improved dramatically if we squatted more, so get your family and friends to do it with you!

It's a demanding exercise, but so worth it. You have to have the physical strength, as well as the heart, to say to the doctor or midwife during labor, "I know what I want, I know what I am doing, and I feel strong."

Georgia, a student who came faithfully to yoga three times a week in her first pregnancy with her daughter, would groan and complain whenever an exercise or meditation went on too long. Then, something changed: "In class while I was whining about having to do our fifteen squats, I suddenly had an image of one of my African sisters alone, squatting in the bush on a cold morning, delivering a child by herself, then walking back to the camp with a baby in her arms. Could it be so hard for me? Since then I not only do them but take them on as a matter of pride, and communion with my history. I have their strength in my blood."

CREATING STAMINA AND POWER

Yoga is how we build our stamina for labor. Go through the discomfort to the other side. If you have to stop, stop. Do not strain. Become sensitive inside yourself to know the difference between stretching and strengthening, and straining. Then, start over. Keep going. Don't run from it, breathe into it. Then when you get to your contractions you don't have to run away because you don't know what to do.

Squat fifteen times. Make sure you do them correctly by squatting with the entire foot on the floor.

- Put your feet parallel to each other, hip-width apart, hands in a prayer position in the center of your chest, and your eyes slightly closed but opened enough for good balance.
- If your heels come off the floor when you come down, double up a blanket and place it beneath your heels.
- At the bottom of the squat, make sure you tip forward, placing your hands on the floor and pushing your buttocks up, then slowly rolling your body up, raising your head last.
- Sweep your arms up over your head, pressing the palms together in a prayer and lowering your hands to your heart.
- Begin again, taking your buttocks each time as low to the earth as they will comfortably go while your entire feet remain on the floor.
- Always use your hands to push up; don't just come up with your legs because that puts too much pressure on your uterus.
- Inhale "Sat" as you raise your arms up above your head, and exhale "Nam" as you bring your hands to the floor.

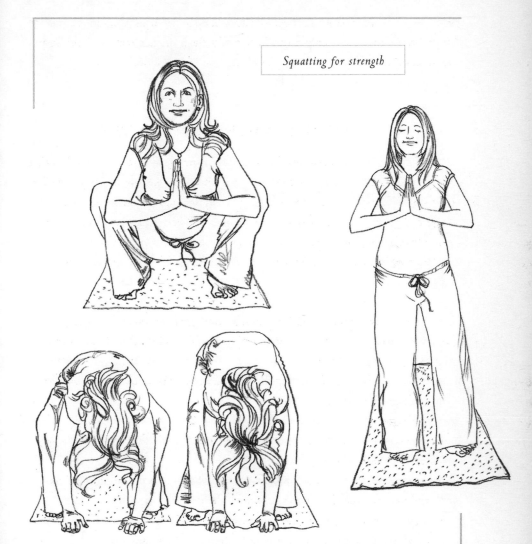

THE
POWER
OF TOUCH

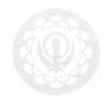

I remember so many people by their touch, don't you? My mother, my father, and even my minister when I was a little girl in church. What I recall most about that beautiful man was the way he would gently take my two little hands and sandwich them inside his very big, soft hands. After fifty-three years I can still feel the warmth of his soul through his hands.

Such is the power of touch. Think of all the knowledge and feelings that can be transmitted instantly just through our skin. Our skin is the largest organ of the body, but that's not something we stop to consider. What comes in through our pores is absorbed into the body. Though most of us think twice about eating or drinking anything loaded with chemicals, too often we slather our skin with consumer, over-the-counter creams and lotions and never give it a second thought.

While you're pregnant keep skin care as wholesome now as you do your diet. Your diet in fact can also help support your changing skin.

- Chinese medicine tells us that by abstaining from eating too many sweets, called "*yin*" foods, we lessen varicose veins.

- Red raspberry leaf herbal tea, sometimes sold under the label "Pregnancy Tea," available at any health food store, tones the uterus. Make a big batch of it, a gallon or so at a time, and store it in the refrigerator. Drink a lot of it every day; it tastes good. Fill a water bottle with it and take it wherever you go. You can't drink too much of it. You'll probably also find that keeping the things you put on your skin and in your mouth as wholesome as you can has some lovely benefits—like softer, more radiant, and supple skin!

One of the best moisturizers is pure almond oil. Buy it in a health food store in many different scents or just plain, and keep it in the bathroom to massage into your entire body before you get into the shower or bath. For your belly, thighs and hips—the places stretch marks love to collect—rub in blackthorn oil (the Dr. Haushka skin care line makes a good one) and the very rich shea butter from the African shea nut.

Above all, keep skin care simple. Reconsider using antiperspirants under your arms. They clog your pores and keep toxins from escaping your body—sweat, like laughter, is a natural release our bodies must have to stay healthy. Instead, use a dab of sweet-smelling lavender oil—it's a natural antibacterial agent known by aromatherapists to create feelings of relaxation and overall well-being and to keep you smelling pretty—or a natural deodorant from the health food store that doesn't contain laurel sulfate or aluminum. Get used to reading ingredient labels. Make it a way of life for you and your family.

No matter what you decide to use on your skin, the most important thing is to use your miraculous power of touch to acquaint yourself with the changes in your body, and with your baby. Keep rubbing your belly. It's a running conversation, because hands have their own language: Your touch can say "How are you? We love you," or it can say, "Come here, let me touch you, let me hold you."

Your belly will be gone soon, but the communication you develop now with your child will stay for your entire life.

PRESCRIPTION FOR GLOWING SKIN

In Russia, pregnant mamas use cold water to stimulate their babies' growth and to release their own fears. In winter, these women, who have grown up in such a frigid climate, break the ice, plunge into the water, and swim in little bikinis, only to come out onto the snow . . . smiling. You don't have to go *that* far to get the benefits, thankfully!

With your hands, massage yourself with almond oil from head to toe. Rub your belly with blackthorn oil. Then, step into a cold shower. Yes, I said a cold shower! It might be challenging at first, but, trust me, you will come to love it, and will actually feel warmer inside! The cold shower will open up your capillaries. When you take a cold shower, blood rushes to the outside to balance the body temperature to protect from the sudden impact of the cold. Massage your belly under the cold water until it becomes warm. That way you give an extra blood supply to the area and that, so say the ancient yogic sages, will give your babies grit, developing great strength. Step out and wrap yourself in a large warmed towel, briskly rubbing yourself to dry. Voilà! Glowing, soft skin, a clear head, and a happy baby.

You may begin with warm water and then go to cold if this is new for you, depending on where you live and what time of year it is. It is best to do it in the morning for a wake-up. Warm, scented baths are perfect for nighttime. You can fill the tub with scents and almond oil, but avoid bubble baths because they take the natural oils out of your skin. Only use natural soap rather than the harsh chemicals of commercial soaps, and then only use it under your arms and in your private parts to avoid stripping your skin. Scrub well all over with natural-bristle brushes or loofahs to help slough off dry layers and reveal new, soft skin! And don't forget those cucumber slices—as you soak, put them on your eyes! Don't forget to light some candles and put on music. You baby is in water, you are in water . . . everything is perfect.

MAKING
A HEALTHY
ENVIRONMENT

It's hard to imagine how asleep and unaware our culture used to be when it came to pollutants in the environment. I remember being a little kid in the 1940s, and how trucks spraying the lethal pesticide DDT would come through the neighborhoods, spraying everywhere for mosquitoes. All the kids in the neighborhood literally followed the trucks, enveloped by a big, black cloud. It didn't smell so good, but we thought it was great fun being in a thick cloud. Our parents didn't think there was any reason to stop us. I think about that now, and I just shudder.

In the Western world we have the luxury of having options to improve our environment. Start now to prepare a home that is more conscious and thoughtful, because what comes into your body also goes into your baby's body. Organic-based cleansers do the job but are gentler on our environment, our hands, our children's clothes, the floors they will soon crawl upon, just to name a few. They can be bought in place of those industrial cleansers we are so used to picking up at the grocery store. Getting water filters for your home's entire plumbing system can reduce or eliminate many of the chemicals that come in through the pipes. So many of us drink bottled water, but think nothing of turning on the shower or sitting in a tub. The truth is that more water is absorbed by your body through your skin when you take a shower than when you drink a glass of water. Don't be shy about taking filtered water to the hospital to bathe your newborn. After the bath, choose clothing and blankets in soft, natural fibers, rather than synthetic, especially for underwear.

You can't create a totally sterile bubble for your baby, nor would you want to. What I am suggesting when I give you this information is to question everything you have taken for granted about your life right now. You have more choices than you imagine in every area of your life, and your family's life. The good news is that wherever there is a challenge, there is an alternative healthy choice.

You don't have to work hard or radically change everything you do to begin to build a home that's healthy and feels good to be in. You don't need money, and you don't need something different than what you already have to make that happen. Just keep your environment clean, and simple, and get things in order if they aren't already—order will be important if only for the fact that, when your child arrives, you won't have the time to look for things! Take your shoes off before entering the house in the Asian fashion. Not only will it help keep things clean, but you'll avoid tracking in potential health threats like lead and pesticides that can cling to shoe soles. Colors, designs, and soft textured materials that babies enjoy are stimulating for everyone, and help create a home filled with good energy. If you don't have them already, add plants and flowers to your home, and art that you enjoy looking at— add anything that helps you remember the miracle of creation that is happening.

EXERCISE FOR ENERGY
AND CIRCULATION

To create new circulation in your home, begin by infusing your own body with more energy and circulation:

- Brace yourself against a wall with your arms out and your palms flat on the wall.
- Lift your weight up onto the ball of your foot, squeezing the muscles of your ankles, your calves and knees, thighs and buttocks.
- Release and lower your weight to the floor slowly so the entire foot is on the floor. Do this twenty-six times, building up to fifty-four if you can. As the circulation increases your legs will burn, guaranteed!

Energy and circulation

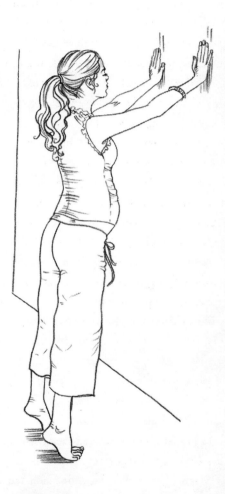

INTIMACY
AND YOUR
PARTNER

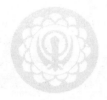

What about sex when you are pregnant? Sandra was a student of mine who couldn't imagine the idea of sex once her belly began to grow. "I feel angry at my husband for wanting to make love," she told me. "I feel like I am as full as I can possibly get. There's no room for sex. All I want to do is yell at him, 'Don't you get what's happening to me? Have some respect!'" Other women feel super-sexy, like fertility goddesses, wanting more than ever to unite with their partner.

There are about as many points of view on the subject from different cultures as there are people on earth. My tradition has historically held that sex is not encouraged after the soul enters at one hundred and twenty days, because the subconscious mind of the baby is being formed and sexual vibrations are too intense. Medically, there's no reason not to have sex in a normal pregnancy with no complications. The love hormone oxytocin that's released during sexual orgasm is the same one that gets labor going—a useful tip to remember at the end of your pregnancy!

What is important at this time is to broaden your definition of "making love." Making love is all about connection and attention and touching and giving, whether or not you actually have intercourse. So often before pregnancy, we use intercourse like the Cliff Notes for intimacy and loving. Now that a new person—your baby—has been added to the configuration, slow down and redefine ways that can offer you both a feeling of closeness and satisfaction.

Dads, if you find yourself out in the cold, I suggest you really get physical—work out hard, go hiking, swimming, do yoga, walk five miles every day with your wife. It will help calm the fires!

Connecting to your partner is a vital element during your pregnancy. Have you noticed there is an entire industry built around babies? Magazines, toys, clothes, furniture . . . you get the idea. And babies are pure sweetness—who can resist wanting to put them at the center of everything? But there is something greater to remember in the midst of all this baby-making. *You are not only creating a child, but a family unit.* It doesn't matter whether that unit is a traditional married unit, or a gay couple, or a single mother who will raise her child in a community of friends. The importance is in the love you have for each other and keeping that sacred.

CREATING DEEPER INTIMACY WITH YOUR PARTNER

True intimacy is cradled in an environment of trust and respect. Tonight, lie together facing each other and take turns telling each other five things you are grateful for about the other person. The examples can be big or small. Don't interrupt each other. Listen from the heart. You might really be surprised; I always am with my husband. Accept and hear the gift of gratitude from each other. Where the heart leads, everything else follows.

Do this every day, and watch what happens!

RECONSIDERING
HOW YOU
WILL DELIVER

"It's a woman's
prerogative
to change
her mind."

I t's funny about human nature. We all tend to act as if things are permanent and unmovable, when in fact everything, even the ground beneath our feet, is moving and rearranging itself constantly. Your approaching labor is no different. A student was forty weeks pregnant, and her due date fell on Monday of the next week. On Thursday she came to class and announced that she had, that morning, changed doctors! "The one I had just didn't feel right," she explained. "I have a much more secure sense with this new doctor." I always say in class that it is never too late to change doctors, and she took that to heart.

We are emerging from what was a kind of "victim" era in America, during which we were able to say, "I couldn't help it" or "What could I do?" or "It was all the doctor's fault." That approach no longer holds. Each of us has to be responsible for being aware of what is affecting our lives. Now that you've done your research about birthing, start to evaluate what you have heard. Who do you trust to give you good guidance? What have you heard that you want to disregard? Take a searching inventory of your relationships. Who can really be there for you and this baby during your labor, and who will not be able to? Making judgments is useless. People simply are where they are in terms of their emotional, spiritual, and intellectual development. Accepting and honoring will give you peace inside yourself and allow you to move on. Now is the time to set your intention about how you will birth and how you are going to live.

If you have made one decision but start to feel scared, maybe that is a wake-up call to explore other options. You have a whole world to explore out there on birthing. If you want to have a home birth, educate yourself about how that is accomplished. Find certified midwives and interview them. Even though home births are as old as the hills, in our country and culture they are reemerging as a popular option. Bring your partner with you while you go talk to a midwife so that you can give him confidence this is not just a whim and that you are going into this responsibly. Give him a reason to trust your knowingness, and then he won't feel obligated to play devil's advocate and second-guess your choice. Know what is right for you and the baby, and he will trust that. Give him *reasons* to trust that.

Contemplate seriously what your capabilities, comfort levels, fears, and strengths are. Knowingness is located not just in your mind. Is there a little voice inside you that would like to explore the option of birthing your child in water? Investigate that. Do you feel comfortable with your doctor? Do you instinctually like him or her just because? I say, look at your doctor's hands. Do they feel good when he or she touches you, are they gentle? Those hands are what bring your baby out. Look into your doctor's eyes. How do you feel? Does your doctor agree with you philosophically? Will he encourage you to reach down and bring your own baby out? Don't content yourself with a doctor or midwife with whom you don't truly resonate. There are so many wonderful, talented, wise, and caring obstetricians and midwives. Keep looking until you find one who will be a champion for your own birth process. *You don't have to explain your feelings to anyone.*

One of the best guides to help you set the environment you want for your birth is a good childbirth education class. Find one outside the hospital where you plan to birth, if possible. Why? You need to hear different points of view. Again, interview the educator to see if she can offer what you need and if you get a good feeling being around her. If you are both in agreement for this soul's arrival, then you won't have to look back and say, "I wish had done this, I wish I had done that." You'll be able to let go and let the experience be what it is.

Set the stage for your birth with great intention and care. Then, in the next prayer, set your intention to remain aware throughout the process and really see what is in front of you. This is different than trying to "control" your birth. I set my intention for Wa's birth, but could not have guessed exactly how it would unfold. It happened at home as I had intended, but the actual experience was far greater than I ever could have predicted.

My due date was February 2, and I couldn't find a birthing center or midwife with whom I felt akin. I had seen several, and they all intimidated me, as that first doctor had all those years ago during my first pregnancy. I kept hearing about a midwife named Shelley Girard, so finally my husband and I met her. And she was perfect. She had a black belt in karate, she was a lay midwife, and she had lived through all the political storms that raged over licensing for midwives and the legality of home births. She'd hung in there through difficult times because she believed in home births, and her calm resolve rubs off on you. I knew she was the one to attend my birth, and my husband felt the same way.

We started looking forward to the prenatal visits. Rather than a five-minute check at some office, we were at her house. She thoroughly checked me and asked detailed questions. We also talked about God, and life—sometimes we would be there for two hours just chatting away. My husband always looked forward to going with me, and you know that's a good sign! Shelley is just a dear heart who gets the bigger picture of who these souls are that are being born.

I was stuck on February 2 as my due date, my labor day, so we were preparing the apartment and getting everything ready. In those days, we were boiling the cloths we would use at the birth. Now you can send away for kits that have everything you need, but back then you had to do all the work yourself.

That morning, my husband and I decided we would go from my house to the

Bodhi Tree, a fabulous metaphysical bookstore that's well known in Los Angeles, which was about three miles from our house. It was a good day for a walk. We were having just a trippy time. I went to the section for astrology to look up what her moon would be in if she were born on the third, because I wasn't feeling anything different. The moon rules the emotions, and looking in the book I found that on the third the moon would be in Aries, a fire sign. I remember sensing very strongly that that wouldn't be it for her. The moon would be in Pisces, because that is more of who this soul is.

All of a sudden, I had to go to the bathroom. I felt like I was in outer space, something had changed! We walked back home—somehow. I remember that I had to stop and lean on my husband for support. When we got home, I just remember sitting in the living room in the rocking chair that we had purchased just for my pregnancy, rocking back and forth, back and forth.

Friends had been coming by to see us all throughout that week to wish us well, because we don't see anyone outside the family in those forty days after birth. I remember a couple came by while I was in the chair, but I didn't feel that I could talk. I was going deep inside. It's funny, the one picture I have of myself pregnant is of me sitting in that chair that afternoon, a glazed, contented look on my face.

That night, we went to bed. Then I woke up around four in the morning, because I felt contractions. This is labor, I just knew, although my water didn't break. As Shelley had said, we got up and walked. I had made a plan to place the baby's first clothes, the blue, yellow, and white cloth of the Divine Mother called Adi Shakti, and a receiving blanket, under the scriptures at the altar of the ashram, so she would get all the blessings. Well, our temple was eight blocks away, a little detail I didn't think much about when I made that plan. But, my mission was to go get those clothes to the altar before the baby came. It was about four thirty in the morning, and I walked all the way to the ashram, with my husband's help. I threw my arms over him while he bent over supporting his arms against his knees. This a great thing to do because you feel totally supported and it allows you to have a good, solid contraction.

I finally got home, somehow. I don't remember much of the walk back because my contractions were coming pretty strong. When we got home, who was walking up to my house but Hari Nam, a friend of mine who is a birth assistant. I hadn't called her or talked to her in days. "I just had a feeling about this," she told me.

Shelley arrived at the house by five thirty. She checked me and I was dilated at six centimeters, meaning there was a little time still. So she and my husband Gurushabd went into the kitchen to talk quietly. The challenge for me was a moment where I felt no one was there for me. I felt, God, where *are* they? No one is doing anything, here I am having a baby and they are having fun! Then something hit me. This experience was meant to be about my relationship to my baby, and that's all. I realized then that Shelley lets you own your own birth. She leaves you alone, she lets you go inside yourself. This was the most empowering moment, because I had to find *me*.

Then it was time for her to check me again. As soon as she took her hand out, I felt I had to push. I just started pushing. I don't remember how long I pushed. I was so in another world. I can't say that it hurt, I can't say that it was excruciating, what I remember was the ring of fire. The ring of fire is that you know this birth is happening. It is like the loop lit on fire in the circus. You have to go through it, and there is no turning back. You know you're almost home when the baby is crowning, then you are to the other side. That sticks with you, that is the sensation you are left with more than anything. After eighteen years I can still sense it. But every birth is different. I don't base this book or the yoga classes on my birth experience. It was one birth. God gifted me this birth, but I can feel in my groin the toughness of a long birth from being with so many women over the years who went through long births and feeling their experience within myself.

Wahe Guru Kaur was born at 6:30 A.M. I only remember holding her. She went right to my breast. We called Yogi Bhajan in Holland, and he was right there as if he knew we would call. I said, "Sir, we have just had a beautiful baby girl. We would be honored to have a name." Then was a big silence, it seemed like a long time, like he traveled the galaxy to retrieve the name that was there for her all along. I can still feel the distance he went. He came back and said, "Wahe Guru Kaur," which means beautiful princess of God's indescribable glory.

Shelley and Hari Nam cleaned up everything, they put on fresh sheets, they cleaned me and Wa, and left me and Gurushabd to lie with our baby. They were gone by 9 A.M. The next morning I got down on the floor with her and did *sadhana*. The beauty of that soft morning cannot be put into words.

Wa's birth was the most exalted day in my whole life. Nothing matches your child's birth, nor your wedding, not the first time you make love. It is when you become a mother, it is the crossing over. This soul comes out of you, and then she is in your arms. Nothing equals it.

MEDITATION FOR INCREASING INTUITION

Strengthen your intuition by coming into Easy Pose and closing your eyes.

- Move your arms as if you are swimming freestyle, extending one, then the other, in constant motion in big circles, elbows pulling the arms above your shoulders.

Increasing intuition (A)

- As you swim imagine yourself in a vast ocean as night is falling and a storm is coming. You can't see the shore, so you use your intuition to determine which way to reach the shore. Project yourself in that direction, and swim vigorously so that the motion will naturally put your breath into rhythm.

- Do this for eleven and a half minutes. You may want to begin at five minutes and work up. Put on music with a good rhythm if you like. Yes, it is hard work, but it is worth every stroke. Keep up!

- Then, come into Baby Pose, putting your forehead to the floor and come onto your knees with your buttocks resting on your heels, relaxing your spine. If Baby Pose doesn't work for you, just bow your head or come lying on your side, or your back if you are still comfortable there. You have made it safely to shore! Feel gratitude in every cell. Stay here for up to seven minutes.

- Inhale deeply and move your spine to loosen it up. Gradually rise and relax.

Increasing intuition (B)

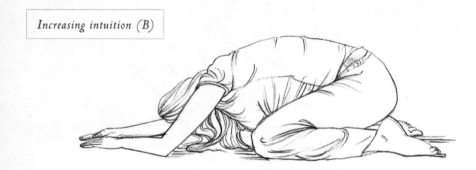

BIRTHING
AT HOME

*"Home
is where
the heart is."*

The beauty of a home birth experience like the one our student Elizabeth shared with me is one of the major reasons I encourage women to consider this option seriously. Elizabeth, like the majority of women who become pregnant, was in good health, had no previous experiences that could put her in a high-risk category, and had no preexisting physical condition that might complicate a natural, vaginal birth. I'll let Elizabeth tell you in her own words about her choices and her experience just as she told them to me:

"I had a friend who had her baby at home, and she started to tell me about it. That was the first time I considered it was possible for me—*me*, a college-educated, professional woman—to do something like that. It was something hippies and women in Third World countries do because they don't have a choice. The yoga I did was also a factor, because it helped me to open my heart to myself as a woman, and helped me create a dialogue with my child prenatally.

"I am really into research, so when I first found out I was pregnant, I researched and researched. I found that the majority of the pregnancy references were slanted to allopathic medicine and only talked about what tests to take and what interventions could be used. The stages of labor were described scientifically, but nobody I read acknowledged this whole other emotional and spiritual side of labor. There is a huge gap in the middle to talk about what labor can be in an emotional way.

"I was trying to figure out whether to go with the hospital. I had found a wonderful doctor who was really laid back who said I could write my own birth ticket in the hospital there with him. My husband and I took a tour of the place. We were seriously considering that option, because we liked the doctor so much. After seeing the hospital I really felt, Thank God the hospital is there, because of the tremendous technology available in our society now. I felt that if I had some risk, I would be in good hands with professionals who are equipped to handle the situation.

"At the same time, I was working with a home birth service. What occurred to me was that if I could create a low-risk pregnancy, my house was probably the safest place for me and the baby, for one because the environment is mine, and I am comfortable there. All this time I was considering where to birth what was foremost in my mind was the point of transition near the final stage of labor, which is where most of the interventions happen. I read a lot about it and talked to other women. I equate it to hiking, when you turn the corner and you can see the top of the mountain and it looks so close, but you really have ten more miles before you're at the top. It's those last ten miles that are killer. You know you can't go back but your body is saying, 'This is ridiculous, I can't do any more.' That was the point I could envision fear digging its heels into me. That fear didn't seem so huge and overwhelming when I considered the experience at home.

"Also, after I had toured the hospital, I just felt that I came away with sickness all over me, germs and stuff. I saw a nurse scrubbing a baby in the nursery, and I understood that it was a totally routine action and that she was accomplishing it fine, but it just looked like she was scrubbing a potato. It made me cry.

"When I said I was going to have a home birth, I totally went against my family. My mother-in-law, my sister-in-law, my mother—at the time they thought, Are you *crazy*? It was scary. People's first thought is that birth is high drama and things happen so fast that if there were a problem there would be no way to get help in time. So I explored that idea and examined the data. I was able to satisfy for my own mind that I was making a logical choice, and could get past that fear that's so present in our society so I could begin to settle down to the question of what I wanted birth to be on a spiritual level.

"A good midwife will tell you that you need to have your health at a certain level or they don't want to take you on. I made getting into great shape a top priority.

"I have been a runner for some time, but I never really got beyond four miles. I decided that birth was like running a marathon. I had to go out and run twenty-six miles for the first time, and I couldn't give up. I thought, what will it take for me to be able to do that? The physical aspect was the most obvious. I could train my body, but I sensed that it would take a real spiritual and emotional side of myself to do this that I had never really developed in myself before. Labor would be just like a race: On the big day, all the people would be looking as I cross the finish line.

"I established a physical plan. I had a chart that listed two columns: one was a 'go for this amount' and another was a 'promise this amount' column. So, say on a Thursday when I got achy and moody, I would look at my chart and it would remind me to keep my promise. I did yoga, swam, and walked in the mountains. It was a great experience, because what emerged from that was this meditative, rather than competitive, approach to exercise. I knew that if I was going to run the marathon I would have to give up a lot about my controlling nature. I can't be present by keeping the nature that I have learned in my life up this point. I would walk early in the morning, and appreciate seeing the moon and sun in the sky at the same time.

"What came to me was the concept of creating my own reality. What does that mean? Visualizing the birth and what it would feel like. I was having this conversation with myself and with my baby daughter as I walked in the morning. The words came to me, and I kept that conversation of what I wanted to create at the birth. That was my mantra.

"The ideal length of labor was a question for me. I didn't know how long or short it was supposed to be. I thought, if it's short maybe it will be too intense; then again, if it's long maybe I'll wear out and won't have enough energy to birth without an intervention. So I said to myself, why don't I just ask for and create the perfect amount of time? I imagined too an experience that would be transforming for everybody who was there, and joyful and earthy and loving. Just this bubble of experience. And that is exactly what happened. Creating my own reality was real. That was so empowering. It was the first time I took this kind of thing on from a real feminine, spiritual place.

"The doctors said my due date was the twenty-seventh, and the ultrasound said it was the seventeenth. But this date popped up in my head as if it were a billboard, that I would give birth on August 20. It's funny that that whole week before she was born, while I kind of knew what month it was, I wasn't thinking about dates. Your brain is just gone when you get to be that pregnant. I didn't realize the connection of the date until afterwards. When I looked, sure enough she had been born on the twentieth. It was one of the most powerful things that has happened to me in my life.

"I don't think about the day I gave birth so much as I think of it as my birth week. On Monday morning I felt different. I just knew things were changing. We went out for breakfast, and I couldn't even concentrate on the conversation. Then I went into the bathroom, and it occurred to me that I could have the baby right there in the bathroom stall! It seemed so imminent. That day I had an appointment with my midwife, who I was seeing every two weeks. I told her about the feeling I had had that morning and she said, 'Do you want me to check you?' Immediately my husband and I said in unison 'No.' We were so outside of the numbers game at that point that it really didn't matter if I knew it was that day or the next or whenever.

"That night, we went to dinner with some friends. I had a big flowing white dress on, and it was summertime so I was tanned, and I was huge. We were sitting at a table outside on the restaurant's patio. Suddenly I had a contraction hit me so hard I couldn't even speak. I got up and went to the bathroom because I just wanted to be by myself. I was afraid someone would ask me a question and I wouldn't be able to talk. At the end of dinner, our friend said, 'Maybe you will have the baby tonight!' A voice welled up inside of me and said confidently, 'No, it's not tonight, but it is soon.'

"The next day, I woke up and was consumed by the idea that I had to finish every task in the world. I called up my brother-in-law and said, 'Remember that thing you needed me to write? I better do it right now.' All of a sudden I needed to have my neck adjusted—when you are in tune with what you need, there is nothing more powerful. So I called my chiropractor and said, 'You have got to adjust me right now.' As soon as I had that adjustment, I just felt this flow of energy through me. My chiropractor told me, 'You are going to have this baby real soon'—she is a mother and had worked on me throughout my pregnancy. My family came over later, we all ate dinner, and they stayed late. I remember walking downstairs to our bedroom thinking, wait, I am bigger than just a few hours ago. I lay on the bed, exhausted. I went to sleep very soundly.

"At two thirty I woke up with a huge contraction. It's important to know that my friend who had first told me about home birth told me this piece of advice: How you choose to describe your feelings is up to you. I had trained my mind during my walks to talk about strong *sensations*, rather than pain. When I had my wisdom teeth taken out, that was painful. This was like a tough workout, which I could relate to from all my physical training. That analogy carried me through.

"When I stood up I had this little trickle down my legs and I thought, 'Oh no, I peed! I must have had to go to the bathroom and that is what woke me.' I went into the bathroom and thought I would have a bowel movement, but, nothing. Then I went back to bed and fell right back to sleep. But then every hour I had the same thing happen. I was in labor, but my brain didn't even register that. I got up at about six thirty and called my mom, and said, 'This might be the day.' She said a mom thing, like, 'Oh honey, are you scared, does it hurt really bad?' And instantly, fear set in. I realized, Wait, I don't need to hear this, so I got off the phone quickly. I realized that as much as I loved her, she could not be in this place with me.

"I lit a candle and started walking back and forth. I felt this intensity. I focused on the candle and all of a sudden I was struck by the need to pray to all women. So

I did. I sat down and I prayed to all women who had ever given birth throughout all time to please come and help me and be with me and support me in this moment. And I am not kidding you, the room filled up with women. First one, then another, and it felt suddenly like I was in a crowded room.

"I got into who I created in my visualization during my walks. That person I had seen giving birth confidently was there, I just needed to step into her. When I did, I stepped out of fear. I could look at my body doing its work. I knew exactly what I needed. I told my husband I needed music, so he put it on. I had thought I would bake cookies on the day of my labor, because I figured it would take a while and I would need something to do. Ha! Yeah, sure. I had a gown I was going to wear picked out, but then no, that wasn't right, and this wasn't right. Nothing felt right. Suddenly I had no clothes on whatsoever. 'Are you sure?' my husband asked. 'Yes, don't put anything on me,' I said. That's how direct and focused I was. I look back and wish I could run the rest of my life like that!

"Three women from my family arrived, and again I was so clear about what I needed—'you, stand here, you, over there.' Of course, I wasn't that articulate at the time. Things were so intense I didn't have a lot of breath to converse. But my family came right in and got into the energy and flow of the situation—after they got over the initial shock of me being naked! I'm the kind of person who usually doesn't like to ask for help, but I realized I needed all this assistance, and was grateful for it. It was so beautiful and so amazing.

"Then the midwife's assistant came at about ten thirty, and I was at eight centimeters. I knew exactly what position I wanted to be in, standing up in some form or other. I felt extreme discomfort when I had to lay down on my back to be checked. I remember thinking, 'You've got to hurry up! There's no way I can be here.' That's something I thought about in regard to a hospital environment: I think because when you have got the fetal monitor on and all the rest of the tubes and straps for all the things they do as a matter of standard procedure, you are not allowed to be in the physical position that you need to be in to let your body do its work the best.

"Sweat was dripping down my big belly and I was watching these undulations, and it was as if I was not even there in a way, another self stepped in, another consciousness. I felt this power in me. All I can describe it as was an instance of truly being in the moment.

"Then the midwife herself arrived, and it was time to push. The assistant went up to get some oil to massage the perineum, but she didn't get that far, because in two pushes, it was over. My daughter was born at eleven forty-five. I had a mirror and was able to see the whole thing. I don't even have the words to say what it was to be present to that. I experienced it as a gift.

"I needed a couple of stitches and it was the most irritating thing, like being pinched—now, *that* was pain. I got up and took a shower, totally exhausted. It takes some time to recover. But I will never forget the sensation of the baby latching on to me for the first time. It was overwhelming, like feeling a miracle happen.

"What I really brought away from the experience is that there is this whole other level of communication and information that flows through me and of me that I can trust. That's what motherhood and childbirth gave me. I tell people I am changed genetically down to the DNA from all this, and from opening myself to it."

MEDITATION FOR COMMITMENT

This will keep your spine strong so you have the backbone and energy to accomplish what you want.

- Come sitting comfortably on the floor in Easy Pose.
- Hold your ankles with both hands and inhale.
- Flex your spine forward and lift your chest up.
- As you exhale, flex your spine backwards, and keep your head level so it doesn't flip-flop with the movement.
- Repeat one hundred and eight times, about three minutes. This will release tension and send energy up your spine. Every vertebra will awaken. You'll feel calmer and more powerful after you do this, ready to take on anything.

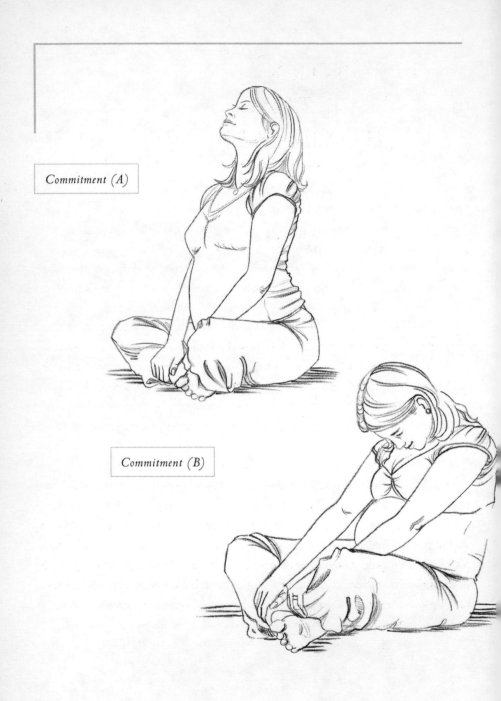

Commitment (A)

Commitment (B)

BORN
AT THE
HOSPITAL

Most women in this country have hospital births, and that choice is a reasonable one, especially if you have any health concerns or a history of difficult births that suggest you might need medical intervention. We are blessed in this country to have at our fingertips the most life-saving technology ever available. Be grateful for that, and let it put into perspective any fears you have about your safety or your baby's.

At the same time, I want you to be aware of the fact that your birth can be and will be as unique and personal as you want it to be, even within a professional, medical framework.

You have a lot of choices you may not be aware you have. You can choose to stay in the bath or the shower during labor if the warm water helps you feel better, for instance. You can choose to touch your baby's head as he emerges and even reach down and pull him out! You can choose to keep your baby with you rather than have him sent to a nursery. I strongly recommend this, because it increases the bond between you and your baby, and eases the shock of his transition into this world. Most of all, what you have to understand is that the medical staff is there to assist you in your work. A doctor cannot bring a baby through the birth canal. That's what you do. *Doctors catch babies; you deliver your baby into the world.* Understand who is helping, and who is doing the work.

Our student Ann's experience of birthing her daughter in the hospital is an example we can all learn from. "I struggled to get pregnant," says Ann, who at age forty-three became pregnant with her daughter. Six years before this successful pregnancy, she and her husband had conceived, but that turned out to be the first of two miscarriages. She then discovered she had endometriosis, a painful inflammation of the uterus lining. After undergoing surgery for that, she experienced an ectopic pregnancy that also failed.

"Then, of course, getting pregnant became our challenge," she says. "I thought it was ironic that we had to go to *in*fertility specialists who were supposed to tell us how to become fertile!" The treatments worked—Ann became pregnant with a baby girl. Throughout the pregnancy she worked closely with her doctor, touring the hospital to get a mental image of where she would be giving birth and to understand what procedures she might face.

But there is an old saying, "If you want to make God laugh, tell him your plans." After yoga on Thursday a week before her official due date, Ann went in to see her doctor for her weekly checkup. Her doctor was concerned that the baby's heartbeat seemed a little slow. "We were just stunned," she recalls.

The decision was made to admit her to the hospital right that minute and to induce labor just to be on the safe side, given the history of difficulties she had faced with pregnancy.

"I went in a little scared and concerned. We had been committed to having as natural a birth as we could, but we threw our plans out the window. I was ready to have a C-section or do whatever was necessary to ensure she would be in no danger. As it turned out we were able to have a vaginal birth," she says. "I had a sensitive doctor, who had both patience and experience. He kept us informed of all the options at every turn.

"Immediately I was given Pitocin and hooked up to an IV for antibiotics, because a test had indicated I had a bacterial infection that sometimes happens in pregnancy. It wasn't my ideal scenario, but I just accepted it. I thought, it just is what it is. To fight against reality would mean spending all my energy fighting a senseless battle. I felt it was up to me to make it work, and to own my own experience."

Still, it was Ann's first time in labor. That, coupled with her worry over the baby and the surprise of being suddenly in the hospital, worked against her. "I realized just how powerful a being I am. Yes, they are giving you a drug that is supposed to work to stimulate labor, but your body is more powerful even than that and can override the effects. They kept giving me more Pitocin. I would peak with hard contractions, but then bottom out. At about six in the morning after I had been doing this for about twelve hours, my doctor broke my water to help the process along. Well, that was no fun, but it was just more awkward than painful. I thought there would be this huge gush of water immediately, but even that took about three hours for the water to really gush out."

Even after all that, Ann's cervix still hadn't dilated past three centimeters, far from the ten centimeters needed for the baby to come out. Her doctor told her that when he returned in a couple of hours they would have to prepare for surgery if nothing had changed. "When I look back at it, it was all because I wasn't mentally ready to go into labor," she says. "My state of mind during that twelve hours was that I really wasn't participating, I was having something done to me. I didn't really know what was going to happen. It was as if something outside was happening to me, it was going to lead the way and I could only wait and follow along. What shifted for me when the doctor said, 'If you have not moved by this afternoon, we will have to talk about our options,' was not my circumstance, but my state of mind. I remember right after the doctor left, my birth assistant went with me into the bathroom and firmly shut the door. 'Listen,' she said, 'Forget about everything else and just concentrate on the end result of having your daughter in your arms. If you need to have the C-section, let's just do it.' Listening to her I realized yes, I want to hold her in my arms, and I have not done all I can to make that happen."

Her husband, meanwhile, had heard what the doctor said. When Ann came out of the bathroom to make her way back to bed, he told her, "Get up and get off of the bed. Let's make this happen!"

Her husband, with the help of her birth assistant and friends, transformed her hospital room into a cocoon for birthing. Candles weren't allowed in the hospital room, so they created soft lighting by bringing in a couple of electric lamps with pink bulbs and pretty shades. "At that point," she recalls, "everybody just kind of stepped back, and the focus fell on us. They gave us space. It was clear to everyone that these parents were going to bring this child in."

With her husband supporting her back and encouraging her, Ann did squats. It was a massive effort after half a day of having powerful contractions caused by the Pitocin, but the two of them got through it. Their favorite tunes from Emmylou Harris, Van Morrison, and Krishna Das played from a portable stereo, and together they did some yoga and danced. As they danced, Ann bent her knees and rocked side to side as her husband supported her, the rocking motion gently helping move the baby down into her pelvis—gravity takes the baby down where it's going, out of you!

"At one point about three hours into it, I said to myself, I have done all I can do. I didn't think I had the energy to do any more. I closed my eyes for a prayer and just said, 'It's out of my hands, God. What will be will be.' I had done all I could do physically, so I went back to bed and concentrated just on breathing and being present. It was like being in the ocean; one wave would come and I would ride to the top of that, then after a moment another wave would come, and I would ride that one out. When the doctor came in he checked me and, miraculously, I had reached about six and a half centimeters.

"At that point I said, okay, I am worn out, give me the drugs! The doctor basically told me without actually saying the words that I was way past the point of no return now, and that an epidural wouldn't serve me now that I had to get ready to push. He did give me a light anesthesia that flattened the edges off the sensations I was having for about an hour. It was brief, but it gave me a chance to rest for about an hour so that I could build my strength back up.

"When the doctor gave the thumbs-up and said, 'It's a go,' the nurse stuck her fists in the air and shouted, 'Yes!' It felt wonderful, like we were a team, they were there with me. By that time, it was about six in the evening, and the doctor said that by eight I would have the baby. He was a little off—I wasn't done until eleven. It took a while for me to find a workable position—I tried squatting, I tried lying on my side, until my birth assistant found in the closet of my hospital room a birthing bar that I could reach up and hold on to. That's what worked for me. My husband was on one side, the nurse of the other, my birth assistant in back and my doctor in front. We got to work. It was intense, no doubt about it, but you get through it."

So after twenty-eight hours of labor, without the aid of an anesthetic, Ann delivered her healthy and beautiful girl, Halle. "It was an experience that shaped our souls and will be with us forever," she says.

A baby is born the way a baby needs to be born, in the exact time, and the exact space.

EASING BACK AND HIP DISCOMFORT

Remember how miraculous it is to be a woman. No man, no matter how strong or sensitive or rich or talented, can make a baby on the inside.

- In a standing position, open your legs as wide as you can while still maintaining a secure sense of balance.
- Form a ninety-degree bend with your elbows, forearms more or less parallel to the floor and extending away from your chest in a relaxed position.

- Now rotate your hips in a plane parallel to the ground at a moderate pace in as large a circle as possible. Move from your hips, not your knees. Keep your knees as straight as possible.
- Work up to three minutes to the left and three minutes to the right.
- This exercise opens your hip area and helps give you the will to fight and not give in. It is believed by yogis that Moses himself used this *kriya* to prepare his people in Egypt to never feel victimized but to experience their own will and strength.

Easing back and hip discomfort

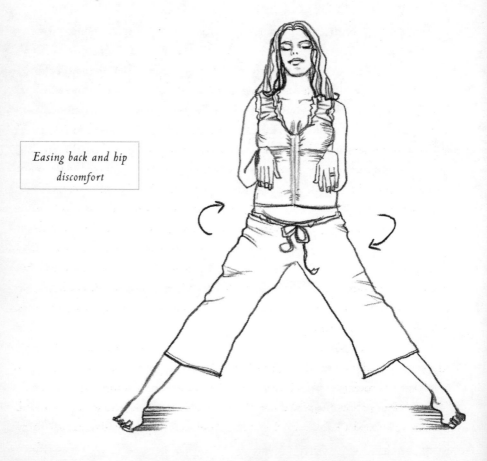

BIRTH BY
C-SECTION

Naomi came in for her first yoga class. At the beginning of every class we usually go around the room for introductions. Each woman tells where she is
delivering and who her doctor or midwife is, and when she is due. She also tells the
area of town where she lives, so if others live close by, they can meet for daily walks
or start a carpool to yoga. This helps build a community and a way for moms to get
to know each other in a big city and build friendships that often last for years after
they graduate from class. When it was Naomi's turn to speak, she announced that
she was two months pregnant and already had her C-section scheduled at a local hospital. I asked her why, thinking that she had some physical issue that would prevent
her from delivering vaginally.

"My mother told me it was the best way to have a baby," she replied. "Why put
the yourself and the baby through such stress? Just bring them out."

I stayed cool, but, while I have heard a lot in my lifetime, I was surprised at how
she was talking about major abdominal surgery as if she were getting a tooth pulled.
As she continued to come to class throughout her pregnancy, she learned many

things she did not know. Naomi ended up having a natural vaginal birth of her daughter Raquel, but her mother continued to call from New York throughout her pregnancy, saying, "I just don't see the point."

The point is this: Appropriate use of technology is important, even vital, but technology as a way to avoid participating in the human experience is not what it's all about. A C-section *when it is not medically necessary* takes you out of the position of owning a transcendent experience into being a spectator in a process that is more about industry than it is about safeguarding health.

Caesarean section has been around nearly as long as childbirth. References are made to it in Greek mythology; Apollo removed Asclepius, the founder of religious medicine, from his mother's belly. Ancient Chinese etchings seem to depict the procedure being performed on living women. I say "living" because from Roman times it was known as a procedure only to be used during the most grave circumstances when a mother was dead or dying, in an attempt to save the child. Some historians say that the term "caesarean" comes from the fact that Roman law under Caesar decreed that all women who were fated for childbirth while deathly ill or after death must be cut open. It could originate from the Latin word *caedare*, meaning "to cut," and the term *caesones*, which applies to babies taken from mothers in postmortem situations. Until the sixteenth century, the procedure was called a "caesarean operation," but that began to change after a doctor named Jacques Guillimeau published a book on midwifery in 1598 in which he used the term "section." Above all, the procedure was a measure of last resort.

In the United States, most statistics say that about one in five babies is born by C-section, about 22 percent of all births. Worldwide C-sections are now being seen as a more "advanced" way to have a birth; reports are that women in Brazil are dismissing vaginal births as primitive—they are unpredictable and can't be scheduled. It is about convenience. Doctors can control births so that their workday falls into a 9-to-5 pattern. Myths that normal birth ruins your sex life push the rate higher as well. The National Health Insurance Corporation of South Korea reports that 43 percent of all births there are by C-section. Good care has come to be equated with paying more, and C-sections are more expensive. In this country the cost is at least twice as high as that for vaginal births.

There is no doubt about it: Having a C-section when there are complications can be a true blessing and a life-saving option for mother and baby. Many women who come to class have had a C-section with a previous birth because of some necessity. They sometimes feel a sense of loss and guilt. They regret that their babies didn't get to stay with them right after they were born, but instead had to be taken to the nursery because babies are usually not allowed in the surgery recovery room. Even if this must happen, don't ponder it too long. You are connected far more than physically to this child who was formed from your body. Just because you cannot be with your baby physically doesn't mean that you can't mentally and emotionally surround her with your white, healing light, reaching out to her soul. That light you project to your baby will surround her and be with her until she can be back in your arms. You are connected for ever and ever. To keep the eternal link, have the baby's father, if possible, stay with her at all times.

The main concern of birthing is that you be conscious of all your choices leading to the moment the baby is in your arms. There are never any guarantees. Fabienne, whose story about her celebration at one hundred and twenty days you read earlier, was one of the most joyful pregnant women I have ever known. While she carried her baby, she did everything "right"—she danced, she sang, she read poetry, she did yoga every day, she ate well, and she meditated, and above all she wanted a natural, drug-free vaginal birth. Yet, when the day of her labor came, she and her husband opted to have a C-section when unforeseen complications arose in her labor. Fabienne and her husband could have chosen to wait the situation out to see if a vaginal birth was still possible, but both of them made the decision that they would feel more secure by opting for the caesarean.

When I first heard that Fabienne had the need for a C-section, I admit I felt angry at God, and confused. "Why, God?" I asked, "What didn't she, of all people, do? This is just not a good deal. What's going on?"

Well, God will answer your questions, but you don't know when, where, or how.

that day, I was in the YMCA locker room after my daily swim. Who should I run into but a woman who took a prenatal class with me eleven years ago. She came over to me and we started talking. I asked her how her son is. "He's such a challenge for me. He is very smart, and very self-willed. I should have known, given the hard time I had birthing him. *He was the author of his birth from minute one.* My second son is totally easy going, and you know he just popped right out."

As I listened, I made a silent prayer and said, "Thank you God for reminding me again." You can always go on till the cows come home worrying over "what ifs"— what if I would have changed doctors? What if I had had a home birth? What if I had not drunk that Diet Coke? That isn't reality, it's being stuck in the delusion that you can control everything. The one and only thing you can know for sure is that children come to earth the way they need to come to earth. As the former student said so eloquently, they are all the authors of their births.

This letter I received from Jerri, a dear student, about her experience during the birth of her second child, wonderfully illustrates the point. Jerri writes:

It's funny how things turn out. Since I did not want another C-section, I only visualized the opposite: a vaginal birth. But after eight hours at the hospital, and given the weird construction of my pelvis (we'll just leave it at that and skip the gory details), my birth attendant and my husband agreed a C-section was in order. I said "NO!" and they let me labor a few more hours. But, my ol' pelvis just couldn't defy the laws of physics. And even though I had a horrendous twenty-four hours after the C-section, I have to look at what is there and not at what is missing. I have a beautiful daughter, and I am once again grateful that I am the holder of one of the most esteemed and honorable positions on earth: I became a mother. Whether one has a vaginal birth, a C-section, or adopts, it's everything that comes afterward that gives true meaning to the word "mother."

A mother. Even after four years of being a mother to my first daughter, I am still learning all that mothering entails. I try to remind myself daily that it is about acknowledging the gifts that I can give. The mother who is great with a colicky baby may not be with a toddler's temper tantrums. And then, the mother who loses her patience at the drop of a hat with a tired, whiny preschooler (me) might be calm through potty training. Sometimes our greatest strength can be the flipside of our greatest weakness. I am learning to celebrate the gifts I bring as a mother. Again, it is to see what is there, rather than what is missing. I see not the little wrong things, but the love. There is such love.

Happy mothering,
Jerri

MEDITATION FOR HEALTH, HEAD TO TOE

Yogis use the following meditation to stimulate every organ in the body to greater health. This breath and arm rotation will energize and stimulate every organ in your body, including your brain:

- In Easy Pose, stretch your arms out to your sides with your palms down, parallel to the ground, and elbows straight.
- On each hand touch your thumb to the mound of your pinkie and then close your fist around your thumb. Keep your elbows straight as you revolve your arms and your fists in backward circles about a foot and a half in diameter.
- Breathe like a cobra with a hissing breath through your nose. Do this for three minutes.

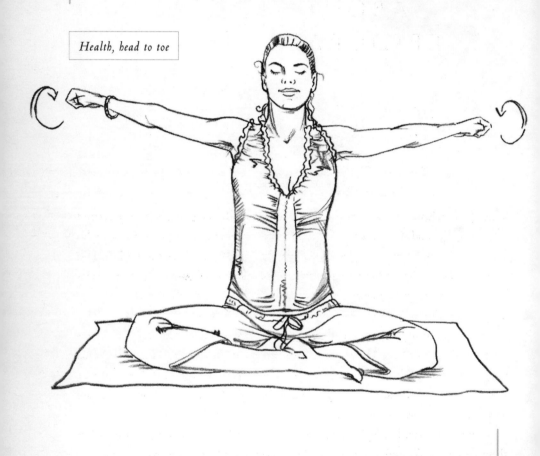

THINGS TO
CONSIDER
ABOUT
EPIDURALS

Holly came to class when she was three months pregnant with her second child, and she was surprised to hear stories from other women in class who had given birth without any anesthesia. For the birth of her first child, Holly had been given an epidural soon after she entered the hospital and she had assumed it was a necessary, standard procedure. "They didn't ask me if I wanted it," she told the class, "and I figured if they were giving it to me, I must need it."

In the past fifty years epidural anesthesia has become a typical—notice I do not say normal—part of the hospital experience. After this anesthesia is injected into the lower part of your back, it numbs the sensations from your trunk down to your pubis. I want you to understand that while this sounds like a good deal, there are always tradeoffs. As the old saying goes, "There are no free lunches."

Epidurals have been a boon for mothers who require C-sections, because it lets them remain awake and aware during the process while being free from the pain of major abdominal surgery. My partner in childbirth education, Davi Kaur, believes that epidurals can be useful for women who have had a history of sexual abuse and find it difficult to connect to the parts of their bodies involved in birth. The epidural can block sensations that might be overwhelming to a woman whose sexuality and femininity have been abused, while still allowing her the ability to deliver and bond with her child in the most natural way possible. Hypnotherapy and meditation during pregnancy can also help to undo and let go of old wounds.

If you can manage the sensations of labor, and if the progress of the birth is within a normal range, I want you to consider that perhaps you won't need an epidural, that the risks of epidural outweigh the temporary benefits. Bring this up with your doctor now, before your due date. Look for evidence-based medicine; the tradition of obstetrics has been opinion-based medicine. That is prudent to know.

There are a few things to think about. Since epidurals interfere with the body's natural production of hormones and neurotransmitters involved in the birth process, they can actually slow labor down. When labor is slowed, doctors give you the artificial form of oxytocin, Pitocin, to jump-start a process that the body is perfectly capable of doing on its own most of the time. Pitocin intensifies contractions. That means when the epidural wears off you are left with harsh contractions and none of the protection against pain provided by your body's own natural opiates. Your body will recover from that, as it will from the backaches that are associated with having a large needle put in your spine, and the ligament and muscle strain that can happen when you can't feel a part of your body that is involved in physical labor.

What I am most concerned about is what cannot be quantified or measured. While an epidural can numb sensations, it can also numb emotion. Have you ever taken a narcotic before? It gives you a feeling of detachment and the sense that you are an observer, not a participant. This same thing happens when a narcotic is introduced to the mother and the baby in the birth process. Some reports suggest that babies whose mother have had epidurals are slower to feed than babies whose mother didn't have epidurals, which makes sense—they enter the world with some of the drug in their system. French researcher Michel Odent, M.D., has noted that the drugs disturb eye-to-eye contact between mother and baby, which is crucial for bonding. When researchers did an experiment with sheep, they noticed that ewes who gave birth with an epidural were completely disinterested in their lambs and wouldn't take care of them. Looking into your baby's eyes releases a flood of oxytocin in your body. If you want to be high on something, be high on the incredible, indescribable love you will feel for your child, which will make every other feeling evaporate.

I think about Holly and how she was automatically given an epidural by the doctor when she got to the hospital. Of course it makes sense that mothers who have no experience of their vastness would want that. When we don't know how to handle pain, we want to run from it. It's an alien concept in our culture to consider that any form of pain can actually be useful. When you don't have techniques to cope with normal pain, or even the experience of being uncomfortable, you will believe something is wrong. If you take the time now to give yourself tools to come to know your body and the power of your mind, so much can be accomplished. Pain can truly be transformed into sensation. Childbirth is a transcendent experience. Going through childbirth without drugs can give you a new sense of power that you never knew existed, giving you a sense of strength that will change the way you approach future challenges. When we feel in charge of our birth experience, we may go into mothering more confidently and make choices that are in the best interest of our children, even if those choices go against the grain of what the rest of society is doing. Discover what the mind and the body are capable of doing. It will be better for your baby, and it will be better for you. I know it for myself and see it in new moms year after year. Having been "checked out" for a long time in the sixties, I prayed to God my daughter would not be like that. That's one of the many reasons I opted for a completely natural childbirth. And what I have been rewarded with is a clear-eyed, heart-centered, level-headed young woman who is strong and confident in who she is.

A student who is an actress, Alex, gave birth to a beautiful girl in the hospital. It was a long labor, her first child, and the doctors suggested an epidural. She refused, and instead created her own pain reliever: With one hand she rubbed her husband's back as he stood next to her so she could draw on his solid strength, and with the other hand she stretched her arm out straight, turning her thumb in a circular motion as we do in yoga class to lose fears and walk through anything that is in front of us. She shut her eyes and rolled them up to her Third Eye point; with every inhale she repeated the sacred syllable "Sat," with every exhale, "Nam."

When the time comes for you to consider an epidural, weigh all the potential benefits and risks, and apply them to your own circumstance. When you put your energy into staying present, everything will work.

PRACTICE FOR OWNING YOUR BIRTH SPACE

Kegel exercises can help you start to own the space in your body from which you will birth: During urination stop and start the flow of urine four to eight times, isolating the muscles of the birth canal from those of the abdominals and the rectum.

This meditation will help you break through fear when it threatens to overwhelm you:

- Sit in Easy Pose, eyes closed, and extend your arms out to your sides, parallel to the ground.
- Close your hands, bringing the fingertips only to the base of your palm, thumbs up.
- Keep your spine straight and your chin slightly tucked.
- Inhale and begin rotating your hands around your wrists, thumbs revolving full circle, up and back to down and back.
- Maintain a tight grip on your fingers and continue for seven to eight minutes with powerful breathing. Start at three minutes if you like. The power of fearlessness will come to you!

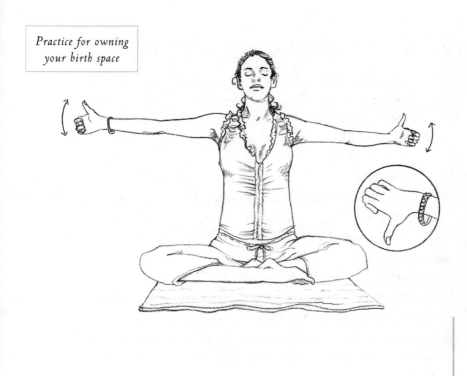

*Practice for owning
your birth space*

WATER
BIRTH

The Greek goddess of Love, Aphrodite, was born from the sea, rising from the foam as it met the smooth, sandy shoreline. That image always captures my imagination, a reminder that our natural feminine strength is the strength of water, yielding but relentless. Motherhood is ruled by the astrological sign of Cancer, a water sign. Its star is the moon, which controls the tides of great oceans just as it does our swells and tides of emotions and feelings.

It's little wonder, then, that this feminine element of water is a perfect medium for birthing. That's true whether you choose to use the warm waters of a bath or shower with warm water pressure on your lower back to ease your contractions and the muscle aches of labor, or to join the small but growing minority of couples using birthing tubs, or to be one of the pioneers who are going to ocean waters to birth their babies among dolphins. I was born under a water sign, Pisces, the fish. Even the sound or just the thought of water makes me feel good. If I had known back in the mid-eighties when I had Wa that it was possible to deliver a baby in water, I would have done it!

French obstetrician and researcher Michel Odent was among the first to advocate birthing in water as the ultimate, gentle introduction of a baby into the world. After all, a baby has just spent the last nine months in a sea of amniotic fluid and is safely attached to the placenta. For his first contact with the world to be the warm, familiar buoyancy of water rather than cold air makes sense. Water is our primary element, composing not only more than 70 percent of our own bodies, but of the planet as well.

In Russia, where infant death rates in hospitals are high and hospital care is renowned to be terrible, there is a movement among women who have begun giving birth at the Black Sea. I show videos filmed there during my couples' workshops, and like everyone in the room I become mesmerized by the incredible beauty of a child leaving the liquid world of the womb to enter his mother's arms. The amazing thing is that there is no surprised look or scrunched-up scowl on babies' faces as they enter the water, because it is, after all, the only landscape they have ever known.

The benefits for you are just as great. Imagine feeling weightless in the water, your skin massaged by it, blood and fluid from birth washed away by it.

OPENING YOUR HEART

This meditation will open your heart and consciousness to new concepts, new possibilities, to freedom:

- Sitting in Easy Pose, put your hands in *gyan mudra,* pressing your index finger to your thumb.
- Begin moving your arms as if you are doing the butterfly stroke swimming through the water. A butterfly stroke means both arms are straight and the movement is back and then up over your head, around and down in front in a full circle motion, pulling the water with cupped hands. This opens the heart, lungs, diaphragm, immune system, and glandular system.
- Breathe deeply and evenly through your nose, and continue for three to five minutes.

STRENGTHENING
YOUR SOUL

Think of pregnancy as boot camp for your soul, a time when you will be conditioning for the challenge of labor and the ongoing challenge of motherhood. The difference between military boot camp and pregnancy boot camp is that one prepares you for opposition (war), and the other prepares you for surrender (love). If you want a birth that can go beyond drugs, if you want a birth where you are present, you have to remap your body and mind. Everybody is afraid; that's not very original. What are you going to do about it? We have to do the clearing.

Make no mistake: Labor is a challenge. It is work. A saying among people in India goes that while a man fights in the open with a sword and spear, a woman battles in the dark behind shut doors.

I sometimes think that what really creates the greatest challenges during labor is that pregnancy comes after years and years of habit about how we relate to our mind and our bodies. Think about the most challenging thing you have ever had to deal with. Where did your mind go? Did you run away? Cry? Freak out? Get angry? All of the above? You need to explore how your mind relates to the challenges you face in everyday life, *because labor is life magnified.* It just is.

Birthing is like climbing Mount Everest. For one, you need a guide you trust and who knows the way, and two, you need to be in condition. There is no magic route, and there is no magic position that will get you through labor, because everyone will experience it differently. There is a magic, and it is found in a woman's ability to focus. There is an old Asian expression that goes, "A focused mind can cut through steel." Think of the martial artist who with the strike of one hand can cut through a stack of bricks. If you have no practice that allows you to develop that focus, you can have a runaway mind, just like the horse who decides to gallop back to the stable, takes the bit in his teeth, and goes.

If you go through labor and you have no idea of the vastness of your spirit, you could be very afraid indeed. You have to have an experience of your vastness before you have to call upon it, just as a tennis player has to practice before playing at Wimbledon. Don't depend only on your mind to get you through—it's not enough. You cannot birth your baby with intellect. Either you are the victim, the prisoner of your mind, or you are the ruler of your mind. Being the ruler is the glory, and the victory, of labor. Having a baby is a lot like being a marathon runner, or an Olympic ice skater, because it's not just a physical process, it is mental and emotional. Making the commitment to have all three of those aspects of your being in the best shape you can will allow your spirit to soar.

Remember, *you are the strongest you have ever been.* You are the most intuitive, you are the most flexible. We live in a culture that has made tremendous leaps in the last hundred years in terms of technology, but too often that has worked to weaken our spirits, weaken our minds, weaken our bodies. We used to chop wood if we wanted fuel to be warm in the winter, now we only have to flip a switch and miraculously we are warm even when a blizzard rages outside our door. Let our pregnancies be the time for us to take our power back and remember again who we are: part of a long, golden lineage of women who have throughout millennia had the strength to survive and thrive. We are strong, we are woman!

The definition of discipline is "training that develops self-control, character." Use that discipline now while you are pregnant, and it will take you through labor and into parenting. It is our responsibility and gift as parents to teach our children, so they will grow up with self-discipline. When they carry it inside themselves, they will not need to search for strength and solutions outside themselves. You have the discipline inside you now; you are Sat Nam, Truth *is* your identity.

We must be flexible to create so much space in our thoughts, our bodies, and our minds, which is exactly what it takes to grow a baby. Never stretch your body so far that you hurt yourself, but do stretch your mind and your spirit further than you thought you could ever go before, because that is exactly what you will be asked to do in your labor and in your life as a mother. The length of that stretch is infinite.

In the sixties, when I first started doing yoga, the big thing was to call women "chicks." We called *ourselves* "chicks." When I started to study Kundalini yoga and meditation, my teacher Yogi Bhajan always reminded us, "You're not chicks. You're eagles, you can soar." And so we are.

MEDITATION TO UNLOCK HIDDEN POWER

The more fearless you become, the more your potential unfolds. With this meditation the universe becomes your mother, and you the child. Call and she will come to your aid:

- Sit in Easy Pose, hands cupped right below your heart center.
- Look into your hands with your eyes about a tenth of the way open.
- Inhale deeply and sing out a long, smooth "Maaaaaa." This is the ancient sound for the creative nurturer of the universe.
- Listen to this sound through your cupped palm.
- Continue for eleven minutes.

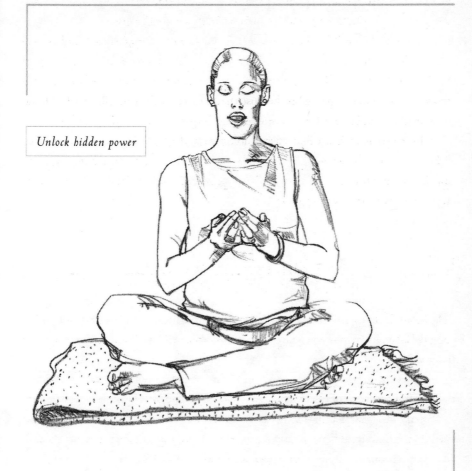

Unlock hidden power

LEARNING
FROM YOUR
DREAMS

> *"In the beginning*
> *was the dream."*
>
> —JOHN O'DONOHUE

You have to have a dream. You cannot just have a hope. If you can't dream at this point, somewhere inside you fear may be acting like a veil, keeping the light of your miracle and mystery from shining through. The story of the soul inside you might be blocked, so you aren't yet seeing how he will come out and manifest in the world.

Often the dreams we have now will be important, although what significance they might have may not make sense until later. I think of the beautiful classic story of Queen Maya of India, the mother of Buddha. For twenty years, the queen had not been able to conceive. Then, one day during the seventh day of the Festival of the Full Moon of Midsummer, she lay down to take a nap and had the strangest dream. She dreamed she was clothed in divine garments, anointed with heavenly perfumes. A splendid white elephant descended from a hill and, after plucking a white lotus with his silvery trunk, he entered the golden mansion where she lay, struck her on the right side and mysteriously entered her chest! She woke up and told her husband, who asked the wise men of his court to explain what the dream meant. They assured her that the dream foretold great joy—that she would have a son who would either be a great king or forsake all power and become the wisest of men. And sure enough, after so many barren years, she found herself pregnant with a son. They named him Siddhartha, "one whose aim is accomplished." Later, he came to be known to millions worldwide as Buddha.

Sometimes you get messages, and you want to discount them. You say to yourself, "Oh, I just saw that in a movie or something." Trust those messages. You are the most intuitive now than you ever have been. How could you not be? You have a soul from the other side inside of you. Two souls in one body! Of course, you have to sift through fears, which also show up in dreams. One student kept having a dream that she gave birth, took the baby home, then couldn't find him. She dreamed she searched her entire house looking for where she had misplaced the baby, only to realize he was in her arms the entire time. Her dream was expressing that worry we all go through when we're first pregnant of "Will I be able to care for my baby?" The answer is yes; all the answers are right in front of you.

I had my own wondrous experience with dreams. As I have mentioned earlier, when Gurushabd and I were first married in 1982, we wanted to have a child, but we didn't know if we could conceive. I had not been pregnant for twenty years, even though I had never used contraception. We married thinking it likely God would not give us children, but then two months after we were married, I remember waking up to do *sadhana*, our morning prayers.

There I was, meditating, but every time I shut my eyes I would see these funny little guys—gnomes, I later found out from someone who knows "that world"— right in front of me. I'd never seen anything like them before, or since. It was as if they were dancing across my forehead, and they were laughing and laughing—I mean, they were laughing so hard they would fall over. They all looked like the character "Happy" from the Disney movie *Snow White and the Seven Dwarfs*. It seemed they were talking to me in between their bouts of hysterical laughter. They were so vivid to me it seemed as if I could just reach out and touch them.

I couldn't make out at first what they were telling me, but eventually they spoke louder until it was as if they were shouting in my ears. "You're going to conceive May 15," they told me. This went on for a couple of days every time I got up to meditate. It was so strange I decided to tell my husband. He surprised me by saying, "Well, instead of doubting them, why don't you just believe them?" I kept seeing them dance across my forehead every morning, until finally I said to them, "Okay, smarty pants, if you know so much, what time will I conceive?" They replied instantly, as if they had just been waiting for me to ask them. "Nine P.M." was all they said, and then I never saw them again. When May 15 rolled around, we were ready, willing, and able! And that's when I conceived my daughter.

There was a woman in my class who went to the beach every day and walked while she was pregnant with her second child. During the walk each day, she envisioned how her birth would be. The picture she had in mind came to her in dreams eventually. It was as if the picture she had etched while walking was filled in with color and texture in her dream. And, guess what, she had exactly that birth, down to the color of the blankets on the bed in the hospital. When you daydream, you are recording it in your baby's psyche, or, then again, maybe your baby is recording it in your psyche.

The famous psychologist Carl Jung believed that a dream, a vision, or an altered state of mind was a "meaningful" coincidence when it happened near some event taking place in the present, immediate past, or near future. He believed this showed there is a "preexistent, immediate knowledge in the unconscious." Yogis had come to the same conclusion . . . about five thousand years earlier.

Sometimes you will be drawn to a certain poem, or a piece of music, perhaps a painting. A work of art can navigate your journey into your subconscious, if you can just release your judgments and go with it. Judgment has a way of extracting joy out of any experience.

Science is able to confirm that a baby in the womb sleeps and wakes, sleeps and wakes. What are the dreams of she who has yet to be born? Maybe the dreams you have now are not yours alone, but visions from dreamtime your baby is sharing with you!

MEDITATION FOR PLEASANT DREAMS

It is said that those who practice this *kriya* (a word meaning "a completed action") have all things they need come to them.

- Sit with a straight spine in a comfortable position and roll your eyes up to your Third Eye point.
- Take your tongue and roll it into a *V* shape with the tip just outside of the lips. Inhale deeply through the rolled tongue, and exhale through your nose. This breath pattern releases obstacles in your mind to allow intuitive truth to come to you.
- Continue this for three to seven minutes.

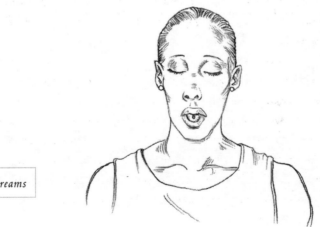

Pleasant dreams

THE
THIRD
TRIMESTER

Put your trust in the bigger space that created us all; that is what brings the baby forward, down, and into your arms.

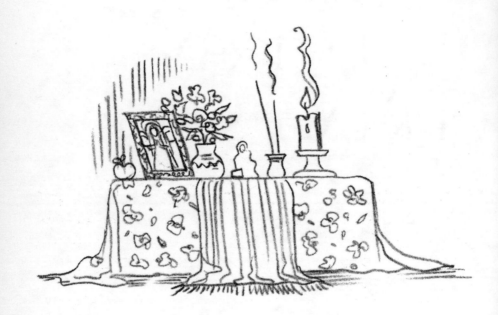

TIME TO
SURRENDER

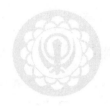

When women first get to class, so many of them have an action plan. They tell me, "While I am pregnant I am going to lift weights and take Pilates and swim and take yoga and do a first-aid class and . . ." I get exhausted just listening to their schedules. What they often end up doing by putting so many demands on themselves is contracting their bodies instead of creating space in their bodies.

Taking care of your fitness is important, but, as with anything, you can go to extremes with that, too. One student was a dancer in the Broadway musical *Cats*. She had been a dancer all her life and had an incredible, lithesome form, straight as an arrow. She wasn't going to let pregnancy compromise her fitness, so she continued with a fairly rigorous training schedule. She did look wonderful, but when it came time for her labor, she ended up having a C-section. Her cervix could not dilate. Perhaps she simply could not release, relax, and let go. Her body, especially her abdominal muscles, was so tight, so taut, that when it came time to let go, maybe she simply didn't know how.

One of the best exercises you can do along with yoga is walk. Just walk! There's an old adage that if a woman walks five miles a day, every day, the baby will just fall out of her when the time is right. When we can walk every day, we definitely do feel stronger and healthier when it comes time to labor. In the very beginning of pregnancy, you sometimes can't bring yourself to do one more thing, and the same is true at the end when the baby has grown so big and you are often carrying so low that moving is awkward. Listen to your body.

Start loosening your grip on the reins of control as you approach that threshold of labor. Release strict concepts of due dates and how you will birth. Each child has a destiny for his birth. Babies are "late"? What an insult to God! Late for their own birthday? There's a month of grace around your due date, two weeks before or two weeks after. Babies are born exactly when they are supposed to be.

You bring your life to your birth, and your life challenges are present at your labor. Are you the kind of person who needs to feel in control? We have this notion that we can control everything. *Put an intention out into the universe, then live in the moment breath by breath.* That is all you need to do, really. When we relax in our lives all things come, when we try to "make" things happen, we tire quickly.

Our shoulders are the place we hold tightness, fear, and stress. In your labor let your birth assistant and your partner know that touching your shoulders would be a good idea to help remind you to release. Now, you may change your mind and say, "Don't touch me" five minutes later, but that's what labor's like—nothing will feel good for the entire time. Notice when someone touches your shoulders that you will find the shoulders automatically lower themselves without your consciously having to think about relaxing them. We don't even know how much tension we hold until it is brought to our attention.

When birthing went out of the home and into hospitals, women started to have a very hard time letting go. Suddenly we are surrounded by strangers poking and prodding and looking at us in the most private of private places. We want to be polite, and modest, and we can't help being worried on some level, "What will they think of me?" We have no context for this experience, it doesn't fit into anything we have known before—laid out flat, naked, fully vulnerable in front of strangers and wanting to have the most sacred, elevated experience of our lives.

Start right now to give up caring what other people think of you. Be yourself.

There is no better place to begin than at birth. When you are in the throes of birthing, you're doing it amidst the blood and mucus and heaven knows what else, and *you don't care*. It is such a liberating feeling. Creation is always messy, like after a strong rainstorm; it defies any attempts to make it neat and clean. One of my students birthed while standing on her tiptoes and squatting. She said later, "I didn't read that in any book!" The truth is you don't know how you will birth, or what will feel right in that moment. When my husband asked me if I wanted to put clothes on after I had my baby, I literally didn't have a clue what he was talking about. "How can you talk about something so irrelevant?" I thought. I wasn't even aware that I didn't have clothes on!

You will never meet a woman who says, "My birth was exactly the same as yours." Start to consider that maybe you don't need to do so much, that maybe all the things you think you absolutely, positively have to have done aren't such a big deal in the long run. Consider too that you are not the ultimate Doer of the universe. We don't need to push a river, the old saying goes. It flows by itself.

MEDITATION FOR TRUSTING AND LETTING GO

This meditation is very powerful. It will help in letting go of fear and resentments, all the mental blocks that hinder the baby's arrival, by trusting and letting go:

- Sit in Easy Pose and raise your arms parallel to the floor with palms facing down.
- Split the fingers of each hand so that the index and middle fingers are together and the ring and pinkie fingers are together, thumbs relaxed.
- Close your eyes and breathe for seven minutes.
- To finish, inhale deeply as you stretch your arms and tighten your whole body. Exhale and repeat this sequence twice more.

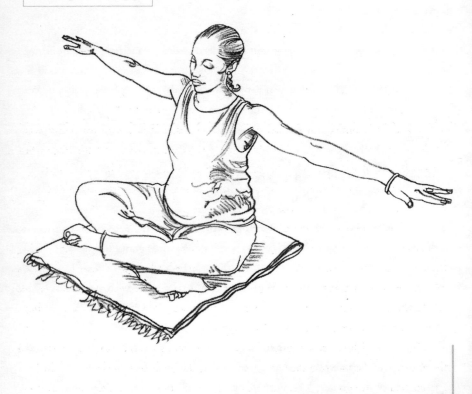

THE ART
OF (NOT)
SLEEPING

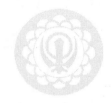

others come to me in their pregnancy, usually in the last trimester, and want me to give them a secret for sleeping through the night at this stage when their bellies have grown so big. There is one notion I offer as comfort: This is preparing you for the time when baby is in your arms. Learning to accept broken sleep, not resist it, will give you more peace of mind.

In these sleepless stretches of time, talk to your child. There is a belief among the ancient ones that if you want to give your child an education, talk to him during the *amirit vela*, from 3 A.M. to 6 A.M. These are the ambrosial hours, when the sun's rays hit the earth at an angle of sixty degrees below the horizon. It is the time when the veil lifts between our conscious mind and the richness of our unconscious. Perhaps babies wake us so we can lift that veil.

There is a Hindu story about this: One day there was an enormous battle, and the enemy had surrounded the forces of Arjuna, the great disciple of Lord Krishna. Arjuna had left to go to a different front. Arjuna's troops were in despair, not knowing how to break the enemy's circle around them, and they asked Lord Krishna, "What can be done?" He told them Arjuna had devised a system of war called chakra, and if someone among the soldiers knew that system, he could lead the troops and fight successfully against the enemy. Just then Arjuna's young son piped up and said, "I know how to do it!" No one could believe it. "How would you know?" they said. He replied, "One day when I was in the womb of my mother, my father was telling her that there is a system that only he knows. She asked, 'What is it?' And as he told her the system of how to form it and manage it, I listened from inside her." The story ends sadly: The son had learned how to advance the troops but not how to retreat because his mother had fallen asleep during the story and his father never finished. In battle he was captured by the enemy and died. If only his mother had been unable to sleep!

We tend to think there is only one way to do anything. Cat naps are the secret. A student who was a professional dancer taught me the "dancer's nap." You either sit or lie down, elevate your feet so that they are propped above the level of your heart, and shut your eyes for fifteen minutes. Remember, cucumber slices on your eyes, lavender oil at your temples and Third Eye point really help relax you. You'll be able to give your body down time in order to restore, but won't fall into such a deep sleep you'll feel groggy when you open your eyes. We are preparing ourselves for that time after we have given birth when we'll need to sleep when our babies sleep.

PEACE SLEEP PRACTICE: WHITE SWAN MEDITATION

Before bed, take a nice, warm, candlelit bath with a few drops of lavender essential oil in the water. After you've dried off, put on a nice cozy robe and come sitting into Easy Pose. This is called the White Swan Meditation, which for eons was among the most sacred and secret meditations used by advanced yogis:

- Make a fist with both hands.
- Put both fists with the backs of your palms toward you, palms away from you six to eight inches in front of your brow point.

- Extend your thumbs and press them together until they become white. You don't need to press hard, just firmly.
- Allow the last joint of the thumb to relax and bend back as much as possible.
- Fix your eyes for a moment on the white tips of your thumbs, then close your eyes and mentally envision the white tips.
- Begin long, deep, and slow breaths, inhaling "Sat," exhaling "Nam."
- Begin by doing this for five minutes, working up to eleven minutes as your focus increases.
- Slip from this meditation into bed and sleep like a baby. Nightie night!

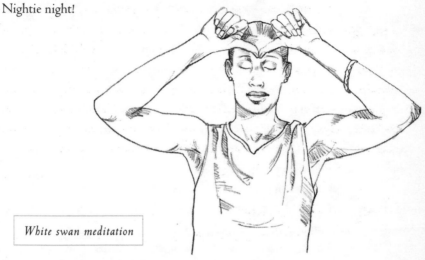

White swan meditation

TRUSTING
YOUR
PARTNER

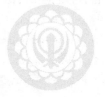

*"Trust is
the fiber of love."*

—YOGI BHAJAN

A student came to our prenatal class, six months pregnant with her second child and deeply troubled. "I am so worried about having this baby." Instantly I thought something was wrong. Had something shown up on a medical test? "Nothing like that," she began to cry. "It's my husband."

Had they broken up? No, not that either. As the time of her labor neared, she was increasingly fearful that, while her husband is a psychiatrist and a man she loves very much, he wouldn't be up to the task of being an effective assistant at her birth. "When our first daughter was born," she told me, "when I went into labor, he brought out his laptop computer and started furiously typing what he was feeling and going through. I couldn't believe it! He was worse than no help, because I felt like I had to care for his feelings while trying to face all my fears about labor. I was miserable!"

And we do make ourselves miserable when we want life to be other than what it is. Seeing clearly and not having a fantasy of your partner as being something other than what he is will help you avert a lot of misplaced anger and disappointment.

Most of all, he is not a woman, at least not in this lifetime. The New York essayist Phillip Lopate once joked in an article describing his experience of his daughter Lilly's birth: "At the moment of nativity, all men are Joseph."

It's not that Naomi's husband didn't love her with all his heart, it's just that he didn't know what to do with the incredible helplessness he felt watching her. Remember, most men don't have an experience of pain as anything other than something being wrong, whereas we women know from our monthly cycles that sometimes pain is just part of a process. The solution for Naomi was simple: For the birth of her second child she hired a doula, a birth assistant whose sole job it would be to support her. That took the pressure off her husband and allowed him to care for their daughter while she labored. That allowed him a way to be a strong father and to support her in the absolute best way he was able.

One student had a husband who grew more and more distant as her belly grew. When she was at the beginning stages of labor, he left the house to go out with his friends, leaving her alone for a little bit. The labor went very fast, much faster than she ever imagined it would. She had to call the midwife because he wasn't home. There were complications with the birth, and the baby had to be taken to the hospital, because she had wet lungs. The mother, having just given birth, couldn't accompany the infant, so the father, who had by then returned home, went to the hospital. Once there, he was overcome. It was his worst fear realized: He was not able to take care of his child. That was the terror that had made him so resistant that he ran away from his responsibility to his laboring wife. The baby quickly recovered, but this was a turning point for this man, who rededicated himself to his marriage and started down a path to self-discovery. I believe to this day that the baby created a reason to engage the father in the life of the family.

Understand that you chose your partner for a reason. He is your polarity; you need that. Don't expect him to be like you—in fact, if he was like you he would probably drive you crazy. He cannot come up with that feminine energy. Let him do what he does well. If the best love your man gives you is making money and providing you with a comfortable life, then hire the best doula or birth assistant you can!

You know, many men can't stand to see blood, either their own or anyone else's. A student who is a hematologist reports that she's lost count of the number of times men have passed out as she draws a blood sample from them. Imagine their primal reaction to the glorious chaos of birth. Often men experience such anxiety at seeing the birth that they experience pain themselves, and they will want you to take drugs to alleviate the pain, which they can only imagine is terrible beyond belief. We have to realize where they are coming from. We are sixteen times more intuitive than they are. Don't resent them for that—they don't have the same characteristics we do. They can only do one thing at a time. Women have the power to think six things at once and juggle three tasks at the same time. That is our vastness, that is their singularity. Love them for their differences!

I know I have said several times by now that you can't read a book to know what it is to be pregnant and give birth, but for most men it's exactly the opposite. They are lost without information. Historically, men have not attended births. This is the first generation of fathers who have been so intimately involved in the process. In our pregnancy couples' workshop I explain to the new dads that they are a new breed of men who are here to help usher in these new souls. Just that alone—babies seeing both Mom and Dad together in their first sight of the world—will build peace on Earth! Sounds too simple, but why not? To be greeted not by someone you have never seen in your life (like the doctor) but by both your parents, and held in their arms, how amazing. How in the world would a man ever pick up a weapon again when his first sight of the Earth is like this? These are the children we call the Aquarian Age babies.

Suggest articles for your man to read, or Internet sites for him to research. Empower your man. Trust your man to provide, and you will give him the strength to provide. Enable him to be excellent. I'll tell you one thing for certain, so many women over the years have said the same thing to me: "My husband was incredible. He really was there for the birth, present, helpful, fearless, and comforting. I was so impressed. I see him with such respectful and awed eyes now."

Assure him that who he is and what he can offer is exactly what you need. Lie around together. Listen to the baby's heartbeat. Have him read to the baby. Sing. Practice foreign languages, tell jokes! Be a family together even now.

PROSPERITY MEDITATION

Ancient texts have been written on just this one meditation for prosperity.

- Come sitting in Easy Pose facing your partner, knees touching.
- Bring your palms in front of you, elbows bent at your sides.
- Begin with the palms facing down, thumbs and the outside of the index fingers striking, then turn them to face up with the outside of your hands striking.
- Keep alternating as you repeat the mantra, "Har, Har, Har," with your tongue pressing to the roof of your mouth right behind your front teeth. Doing this for seven minutes brings abundance on all levels!

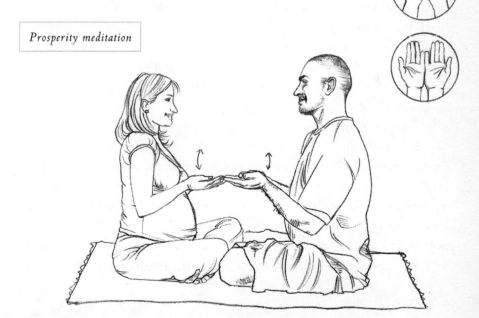

Prosperity meditation

REDEFINE
THE IDEA
OF PAIN

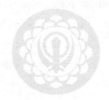

For our entire lives up to this point, the word "pain" has been associated with something wrong, with injury to our bodies. Labor is not injury; a woman's body is designed to accommodate it! We need to change our vocabulary. Rather than saying the "pain" of labor, we can say "sensation." Okay, "strong sensation." The word "sensation," on the other hand, means, "Pay attention! Something important is happening! Something so right is taking place!"

I often think that much of our perception of childbirth as a process of horrible, unbearable pain comes from the fact that, in this country, we most often go to a hospital to give birth, an institution that functions to heal and care for the sick and injured. Medicine tends to approach birth as a potential catastrophe, not as a likely joyful event. When you think about it, a pregnant woman is the only patient routinely checked into the hospital when something is *right* with them, not when something is wrong!

What causes the "pain" of labor? The ligaments of the uterus are stretching, the uterus itself and the surrounding muscles are stretching, and the child is pressing on your cervix, the lower vertebrae of your back, and the birth canal. If you are having a conversation with yourself that these sensations are painful, the longer you have that conversation with yourself, the longer you block the possibility for any other experience to occur. Think about it this way: We all need to remember to differentiate "pain" from "challenge." Pain leads to more pain, challenge leads to victory.

Labor will be overwhelming to you if you think about it as one long, unending, constant pain. That isn't what it is. Rather than think about ways to distract yourself from pain, dive right into the middle of the sensation and welcome it, because with every contraction you are that much closer to holding your baby in your arms. Go deep within yourself and find that meditative mind; what you will find is a way to feel each discrete moment. In one instant there will be pain, and in another there will be sensation—a big difference.

Think of yourself as being out on the end of a diving board. There's the diving board, and below you is the water. In between the moment when your toes leave the rough surface of the board and the moment when the cool water hits your skin, there is an emptiness in the space between the two. Find those spaces in your labor by burrowing deep within yourself. How? With breath, inhaling the sound "Sat," exhaling the sound "Nam."

How we think about pain actually influences how we feel it. If you say to yourself "This is horrible, I can't stand it," there's a good chance that whatever you're going through will feel a whole lot worse than if you believed the feeling wasn't so dire. If our previous conditioning is to associate pain with danger, then we are more susceptible to suggestions that labor is dangerous and requires external relief in the form of drugs. When we learn to associate the feelings of labor as signals that herald a powerful transition, it's astounding what we can accomplish.

How our culture at large views pain also influences our perception of it. If we get messages that all pain is to be avoided, well, guess what? These cultural attitudes are translated into personal fears, doubts, and our ability to manage labor—manage our lives, for that matter. Our pharmaceutical companies are built around this idea.

We are part of this whole thing, this universe. If you can connect to that, you can connect to this instrument that is your body, and you can connect to your birth. If you meditate on this more than anything else, it will change you not only during your pregnancy, but for your life. Put your trust in the bigger space that created us all; that trust is what brings the baby down, out, and into your arms.

MEDITATION FOR PREPARING FOR BIRTH:

LEAVING THE FEAR AND WELCOMING THE CHALLENGE

This will clear the worry out of your chest, heart, and lungs, and replace it with love and optimism.

- Extend your arms straight out to your sides with your palms facing out as if you're a traffic police officer holding back cars at an intersection.
- Inhale as you raise your arms up over your head, creating an arc; your palms cross over and slightly in front of your head, but do not touch.
- Exhale your arms down. As you exhale, lower your arms to their original position. On the next inhale raise your arms again but cross the palms over and slightly behind that top of your head. Continue this for two minutes, work up to seven minutes.

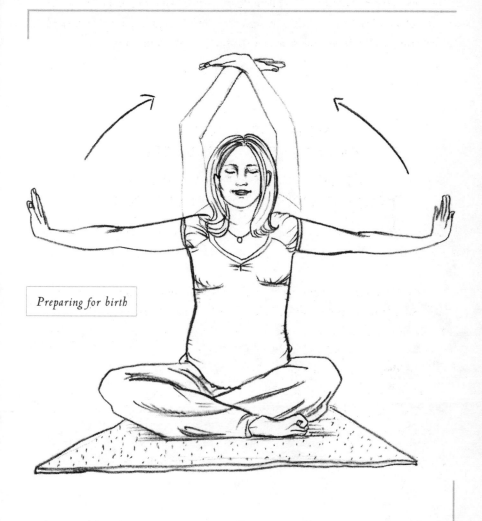

Preparing for birth

PREGNANT PAUSE: WAITING FOR THE BIRTH

Labor is like the weather: unpredictable.

Due dates are imaginary numbers not created by God. It's something that we get caught on, but your body will do labor when it's ready. Our babies are born at the certain time and the certain place, otherwise there would be no order to the universe. Think of it like a summer sunset: Do we stand out of our houses at dusk each day and wonder, Will the sun go down tonight? Of course we don't! We know it will, we know where it will, and we know what time it will. There is a divine order just as there is a divine order when it is time for souls to be ushered to the earth.

When that soul emerges, when that first breath is taken, the configuration of the stars and the heavens is just so. The Tibetans believe that regardless of the due date, a baby won't come forward into the world until the star under which it is destined to be born is shining. The universe is not randomly ordered, but we randomly pick these things called due dates. When we get hung up on these due dates we set ourselves up for disappointment, fear sets in, as well as a feeling of failure or "Is there something wrong?" We think about what more we can do to get this labor started rather than letting the labor come to us.

Babies have a way of arriving by one means or another when they want to. A student came to class when she was due in five days. She gave me a whole laundry list of things she had to do before she could turn her attention to her impending labor—graphics on the computer for work, furniture buying, check book balancing, and so on. I said, "When can you be done?"

"Tomorrow," she replied.

"Okay," I told her, "be done. This baby is not going to come—I'll put money on it, I have been around long enough—until you meet the frequency of this baby. That means you have to slow down, space out, sleep, take a walk, get into that realm. The baby will wait until you get into that realm. They want to come out when you are not too busy for them."

I tell mothers who are near their labor, "You've got the glazed look." I even sometimes suggest they stop driving and let other people run their errands. We know the baby is coming when you get that look. You're like a pumpkin lit by a candle from the inside. When the candle inside is lit, the plain pumpkin is transformed into something spectacular.

We are always looking for a schedule—let that fly out the window. Just be there for yourself and for your baby inside you who is preparing for his birth journey. I want you to think of a list of "Things NOT to Do." Think, How much can I relax? Who cares if you have slept twelve hours but need to sleep more? Sometimes you are so tired these last months; at other times you burst with energy. You have to get used to the ebbs and the flows, because these little ones are preparing you for motherhood. That's the way it is—sometimes your babies eat a lot, sometimes not so much. Sometimes they want to be held, sometimes they want to just lie still and space out. Sometimes they sleep, sometimes they don't—you get the picture. Pregnancy is practice for what you will be doing for the next years to come.

Talk to your child. You are mentally, spiritually, and physically linked; that is why there is nothing stronger than your own prayer for this child. Whenever you want to be with your baby, roll your eyes up to your Third Eye point, which corresponds to your pituitary gland, called the master gland because it regulates hormones. That is your direct line to the womb. If you get quiet enough, you will know what your baby is thinking and feeling.

Sex and walking—not necessarily in that order!—are known to help labor. If you really want to get labor going, I say try hanging out with babies and children. Hold them, play, and laugh with them. They get the oxytocin pumping in your system, and it is as if they are calling to your child, reassuring him, "It's fine out here! Come on out! Come play with us!" We had a dinner party for my husband's birthday some years ago. One due mama attended, and there were four or five infants and a group of toddlers there. I put all the children in her arms. It wasn't hard—they were so attracted to being around her all night. She went home and, what happened? She went into labor!

MEDITATION WHILE WAITING FOR BABY

You need to get your partner or a good friend who will be at your birth to do this *venus kriya* with you:

- Sit facing each other, knees touching, and look into each other's eyes.
- Put your palms together, fingers up with your partner's.
- As you push each other's palms back and forth, alternate hands like paddling a boat. Sing as you rock from side to side:

  Row row row your boat
  Gently down the stream
  Merrily merrily merrily merrily
  Life is but a dream

- Listen to the words as you sing them—they're reminding you to go with the flow.
- Do this for three to five minutes. Have fun and laugh! Remember, your baby is hearing the words, too.

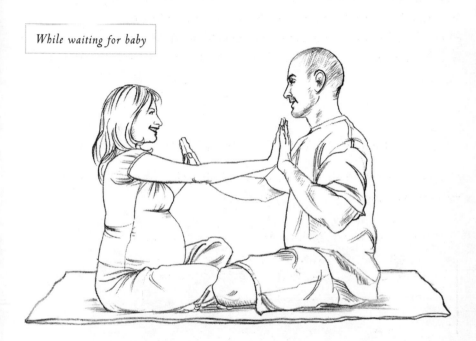

BIRTH . . .

Your spirit as a woman
has all the knowledge
and power you need
to give birth
and to nurture
your baby.

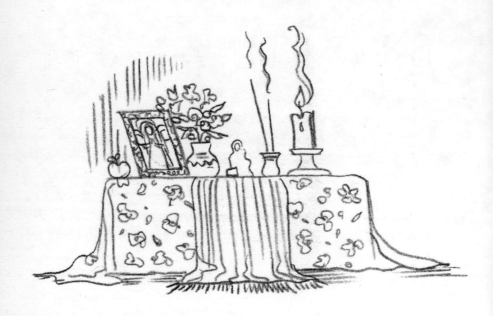

WHAT
LABORING
WOMEN NEED

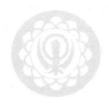

Every year at Christmas, Christians tell one of the greatest birth stories ever known about the young woman named Mary. On a starry night in the quiet of a manger in Bethlehem, amid the animals, Mary delivered Jesus, whose message of love and peace continues to inspire. The story of Buddha's arrival is also very inspiring. His mother, Queen Maya, was said to be in the Lumbini Garden and, reaching up to pluck a beautiful bough of blossoms, she began her labor. She was still standing under the blossoming tree when her attendants found her with a baby boy held to her breast.

You'll notice the one thing these divine births have in common is that their mothers were nestled away in a private, peaceful, and natural place, away from prying eyes and strange faces. These births from thousands of years ago echo modern researchers' findings about what laboring women still need today.

In labor, we change our state of consciousness. In labor, the most active part of our brains includes the pituitary gland—remember, that is the Third Eye point—and the hypothalamus, which are also the oldest, deepest parts of our brains that we share with all other mammals. People who have been around women in labor can tell you it seems as if they are on another planet—and they have to be, in order to reduce the influence of the brain's neocortex. Things that stop labor, like adrenaline release, come from the neocortex, the so-called intellectual part of the brain. The basic need of labor is to be protected against any stimulation of the neocortex.

So what stimulates? Language, for one—like being asked questions. Bright lights are another stimulator, as is the feeling of being observed. That's why I say we must honor the birth experience. Consider leaving your video cameras at home, question the absolute need for a fetal monitor if you have had a healthy pregnancy and are proceeding normally, turn the lights down and shut your eyes. And pray. At this time you need only to be yourself beyond your personality, be private and humble, grateful to be part of this wonder called the human experience.

If you are at home, it is a whole other world. You can light candles, play music, go into the kitchen, walk out to the backyard and look up at the sky, smell the roses in the garden!

You can't read enough books to know what your labor is going to be like. The best book you can read is written inside you. The more you read it, and the more you get to know it, the more you will move powerfully into birth. Your body is going to tell you, "Relax, we know what we're doing."

USING MOTHER EARTH ENERGY
MEDITATION

- Sit in a comfortable position on the floor or outdoors on the Earth and roll your eyes upward. Think of pulling energy from Mother Earth up your spine as you inhale.
- As you exhale, take that energy down through your spine and back to the earth once more.
- Do this for seven minutes as you hear the sound "Sat" on the inhale and "Nam" on the exhale.

- Wrap your arms around your belly, your baby's home. Start to feel how Mother Earth holds the space for you and the soul within you, and how she will support you and uplift you if you but call upon her.

As I write this, I am crossing the Rio Grande Valley in New Mexico, going to the Summer Solstice Celebration. I feel Her so very much. The stars shine so bright above. I walk in Her moonlight and feel Her vastness beneath my feet, feeling at this moment that anything is possible. Newspaper headlines, CNN, all worldly trauma is gone. This meditation takes you there whether you are in New York City or Tucumcari, New Mexico!

WHO
ATTENDS
THE BIRTH?

It doesn't take a village to have a baby. Now, *raising* a child might be another matter, but for your birth, surround yourself with those people who won't feed into fear or transfer it to you. Protect yourself and your child from needless tension during this time by not inviting everyone to the party.

At the point when you are tired and aching and you doubt your own might, when you are so near to losing your truth and your confidence, you have to look to the faces of people who can and will hold your truth and your confidence for you. I once was at a birth where all the mother's relatives showed up—her mother, sisters, brothers, aunts, and a few cousins. That can work, but in this case they came as spectators, and the laboring mother fell into the role of hostess, trying to make sure everyone was comfortable and had food and drinks. It distracted her from her birth experience, and only when we requested that they step out into the waiting room was she able to get down to the business of birthing and seriously started to dilate.

Labor support can make all the difference in your experience. A doula is an important figure, because she is your advocate. She can help hold the sacred space, and tend to the flame of your commitment when it flickers. *"Doula"* is a Greek word that has come to mean "she who mothers the mother." The presence of a doula can shorten labor time, decrease the amount of pain medication or eliminate it entirely, and significantly reduce the caesarean rate. A letter I recently received from a student, Cynthia, is a good reminder. She writes:

"... I cannot say enough about how wonderful Carmen is as a doula. I was in labor for thirty-eight hours, the reason being that my body liked to take its time dilating. Believe it or not, it would have been twice as long if it weren't for Carmen. She is licensed to do internal examinations for her clients in their homes. Because of this ability she was actually able to massage my cervix to the next centimeter, thereby helping my body along. We know in hindsight how valuable this technique was because when I reached six centimeters and went to the hospital, things changed. But, because of my doctor's great prenatal care and Carmen's support during the delivery, I had the birth of my dreams. I wouldn't trade one hour of labor for anything in the world. Each step of the way taught me so much about myself, and each step was necessary in the big scheme of things."

I was giving a seminar in New York when a student came up to me. She had given birth to her baby about a year and a half earlier. As she told me her birth story, it echoed what seems to happen a lot these days. When she went into the hospital, she did not have anyone with her who could act as her advocate. She went in when her baby was only five days "overdue," as the doctors said. Remember that two weeks before or two weeks after your due date is still considered on time. Babies have that month of time to come out when they need to come out.

Anyway, she went in for a sonogram, and they found that her amniotic fluid was low, so they would not release her from the hospital, and they induced her right then and there. She went from Pitocin to an epidural, to eventually having a C-section. If you are ever told that your amniotic fluid is low, *but your baby is not in stress*, go home and drink a lot of water and eat juicy fruit and cucumbers and see what happens. In some cases, you can get that fluid back up again. Why be induced if you don't need to? But this young mother just didn't know.

Many times with a hospital birth questions are asked during labor by the hospital staff. You need to begin the process of spiraling inward to reach that ancient, precognitive part of your brain in order to do the work of birthing, and every time you are brought back up to the surface, as it were, the process is disturbed. Having someone with you on whom you can rely to be your spokesperson is an excellent idea. To make informed choices during labor, questions such as these need to asked:

- Why is this intervention being considered?
- What do you hope to accomplish by doing this?
- What will happen to my baby and me if we do this?
- What will happen if we wait awhile before deciding?
- What alternatives can be considered?
- What will happen if I choose not to do it?

Someone who is informed and is looking out for your best interest is so vital to help you ask the questions and reason out the answers. This is clearly where doulas can come in. One of the best phrases to remember, unless you are in a clear emergency, is "Doctor, we need a little time to talk privately."

EXERCISE FOR CASTING OUT DOUBT

- Stand, and then place your hands firmly on your thighs above your knees, keeping them slightly bent.
- Exhale and bring your chin to your chest, tucking in your tailbone. This is called Standing Cat Pose.
- Then inhale, raise your head and tip your pelvis up, creating a sway in your back only as much as is comfortable. This is called Cow Pose.
- Alternate these poses for a minute, or as feels good.
- Then, begin to grind your pelvis in a circular motion clockwise.

• Do this for three minutes; reverse and continue, keeping your knees bent and the pressure off your body. It must feel good.

This is a posture to take a few minutes to clear your mind and receive clarity, passing through the valley of doubt to clarity. Keep your eyes closed and focused upward if you can and still feel balanced. Keep them open if you can't.

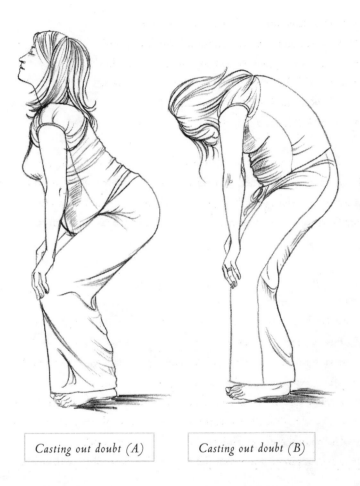

Casting out doubt (A)   *Casting out doubt (B)*

LABOR

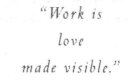

*"Work is
love
made visible."*

— KAHLIL GIBRAN

Everybody seems to be quite serious about everything in the pregnancy world. Is it just Los Angeles? I don't think so. Everybody wants to be perfectly enlightened, and they work really hard. You want to have a perfect birth, and a perfect child. Just the word "labor" makes people serious. Receive birth with joy in your heart—your baby will soon be in your arms! At our pregnancy workshops with the moms and dads, we include yoga meditations along with singing, eating, dancing, and laughing to allow everyone to open up and celebrate life and this wonderful adventure called having a child.

Don't wish for labor to be over and done. You'll miss living the moment right now. We never really live when we're always jumping ahead or stepping behind.

Remember Ann in her hospital room? Dance, walk, do squats if you like with your partner's loving aid. It is all about spiraling inward to get in tune with the sensations in your body. Hug, play, and talk softly and intimately with each other. Kiss! The same energy that got the baby in is the energy that gets the baby out. Let the center of your dance be your belly. You are bringing this soul only one foot along down the birth canal in his lifetime journey! "Understand that every time a contraction comes, it's bringing the baby that much closer to your arms," my partner Davi always reminds parents in the childbirth classes.

When each contraction is over, come back to your breath. There is a sweet but very powerful little chant we recite to help our babies along their way. It's something you can do throughout your pregnancy. It goes like this—think of it as a football cheer with you as the cheerleader and your baby as the star player!

> *Head down!*
> *Chin tucked!*
> *Back to belly!*
> *Arms down!*
> *Yeah Baby!*
> *Yeah Baby!*

In the middle of a challenge or a storm, the answer is always here if you can get quiet enough. Sometimes someone will say something that seems to be just a random or inconsequential remark, but it will lead you to another thought, and in that thought you may realize what you needed to understand. The random remark was a gift, reminding you of what you already know. This happened the other day while I was talking to my older brother on the phone. We were reminiscing about all the people in our lives who helped us along the way. There is no one we can talk to quite like old, old friends and siblings about our past, because no one can remember back through our lives as they can. Then my brother said, "It's amazing how someone can just be talking casually, but what they say—one line, one thought, a word—can change your life, but they may never know it. It's like God speaks through us all in a wondrous way. I guess that is what the power of the word is; what the word of God is."

In labor, call upon something bigger than you. If the idea of God is a challenge for you, call upon all the souls of women before you in all time to help bring your baby forth into this world. Realize the infinity in the collective strength of women.

There is a true sisterhood in that. A famous Zen koan asks, "That girl over there, is she the younger or older sister?" The question is meant to lead you to the understanding that in the most absolute sense, there is no "over there," no separation between yourself and another woman, no space and time, just one infinite continuum of experience. Remember the story of Elizabeth, who called upon the strength of all women throughout space and time who had ever given birth to help her in her moment of need, and how she felt the room fill with souls and heard them say, "Yes you can, yes you can." Call upon all saints and sages with whom you feel affinity to also come forward.

The Third Eye point we refer to in yoga corresponds directly to your body's pituitary gland, which releases oxytocin. Oxytocin in turn makes the uterus contract. Your brain is constantly regulating labor as it takes in a number of different messages, including clues about your emotional state. Fear and anxiety shut down the flow of oxytocin, and can make labor more difficult and can even stop it. Lavender and neroli (orange blossom essence) are relaxing essential oils that can help you at your birth. Try a couple drops on a cloth or tissue, hold it to your nose and see if you like the scent. If you do, it can bring up positive associations and help you relax in labor. No one knows the exact mechanism that starts labor. The ancient texts suggest that your baby actually meditates on you, the mother, like knocking on a locked door: "*Mataji* (Beloved Mother), I am ready to come now!"

Lose all thought. Go beyond counting, how long a contraction was, how many centimeters, how many hours you've been in labor, if you've slept. Most of us don't know how to handle pain, so we want to run from it. Our minds get stuck on the last contraction; that's an event that has already happened, it's part of the past. *Experience it, and let it go.* Your job is to ride each wave, the one right in front of you, just like surfing. If you jump ahead or fall behind the wave you fall off the surfboard, and you become afraid. If you stay in the middle you will not be afraid because you will be present to the experience that is happening. Ride one wave at a time, not looking back, not looking forward. That is what I mean when I tell you to create a meditative mind.

The biggest word is *surrender*—birthing is like life, there are no guarantees. Can you surrender to each breath, to each contraction, to the Creator who created you and this baby? Lean on that Creator to bring the baby out. You are not the one, ultimately, who made this baby. That power belongs to the same power that creates stars from dust. Yet at the same time, you are not separate from that power. We say, "God and me, me and God, are One." This is the time to fill the room with all the mothers, saints, and sages that have gone before you. Change your emotion (namely, fear) to devotion. Now is the time for patience. Remember, patience pays.

MEDITATION FOR POWERFUL FOCUS

- Sit in Easy Pose.
- Stretch your arms out to your sides and up at sixty degrees, palms faced inward and fingers pointing up.
- Sing "God and me, me and God, are one" for three minutes with your hands over your belly

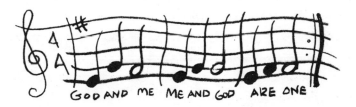

"God and Me" melody bar

THE
SECRET OF
MOTHERING

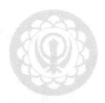

I once asked a very wise saint in India, "What is the meaning of the word sacrifice?"

He said, "It is simple. It is when you take yourself out of the middle of the circle."

When you go into labor, you take yourself out of the middle of your circle of existence, and you place your baby into it. This light so bright that the love for this child will lift you out of the middle into celebration. Let your "self" fall away and become something greater than what you have ever imagined possible.

"For me," says our student and friend Seannie, "giving birth was an act of surrender. Suddenly I was no longer the center of the universe." She is the mother of three, all born at home. Her life was so transformed from her births that she became a doula and is training to become a midwife. Her passion to help other women is such an inspiration to me.

In the moment of birth, mothers are born as mothers, fathers are born as fathers, families are born as families.

MOVING
THROUGH
FEAR

When fear overwhelms truth and love, we call it pain. Our spirit as women has all the knowledge and power we need to give birth and to nurture our babies. It is in our genetic coding. It has been there since the beginning of time. You can trust its wisdom.

If we can stay focused at the Third Eye point during labor, we will have all the information we need. Those voices on the outside of you are only making a guess about what is happening. How can they know truly what is inside? That is your province. Listen to them when it serves you; however, you are the ultimate authority. Travel down the steps into your mind's eye, and stay there. That is the place of your power. Either you are a prisoner of your mind and your fears, or you're the ruler of your mind. As you'll see, that's the glory, and the victory, of labor: to be the ruler, the queen of your mind.

Ask your labor assistant to always help bring you back to your own center of power, not join you in your fear. Ask that of everyone in the room helping you.

Where there is love, there is no fear. Be in a clear space of possibility where you love your labor because it is the process that allows your child to come out into the world. Every time you feel grateful for something, it counters a fear. In other words, if you start getting caught in that loop of fear—"this is too much, I can't do this, it hurts too much . . ."—just come back to the simple process of breath moving up and down your spine, "Sat" on the inhale and "Nam" on the exhale silently or out loud, and draw your attention to something for which you are thankful. It can be the same thing over and over. Fear cannot live in thankfulness.

There are very good physiological reasons for moving through fear. One, because it is known to contribute to the experience of more intense pain during labor. Imagine a little cottontail rabbit: If the mother feels safe and secure in her burrow while she is giving birth, there will be low levels of adrenaline in her bloodstream. Then, say a fox comes and sticks his head in the burrow while she is in labor. That will cause her adrenaline to rise and stall the labor, in case she should need to fight the fox or flee to the safety of another burrow.

The uterus is the only muscle in your body that has two opposing muscle groups. One contracts and opens the cervix, and the other closes and tighten the cervix to stop labor. When a birthing mother becomes afraid, adrenaline creates the flight-or-fight response and tightens the cervix while at the same time the uterus continues to push the baby's head down with each contraction. The result is the very real pain of two powerful muscle groups pulling in opposite directions.

What increases fear in us? The fantasy of the unknown. But birth is not unknown; it has been progressing the same way for millions of years, among humans and animals alike. Trust that you are not going into the unknown. The territory of birth that lies in front of you can be navigated, even more so if you have taken the time in your pregnancy to come to know yourself.

All the meditation you have done is bringing the breath back to you. Once you understand "Sat Nam," Truth Is My Identity, you take the process out of drugs and doctors and into the realm of knowing. There are mothers inside you, the spirits of those that have come before you, who know. Ancient teachings tell us we have been here 8.4 million lifetimes. Can you even begin to imagine how many children you have birthed? And still we think we don't know how. When you see God in all, then you are not afraid of anything. That is the true yoga, dwelling in Infinity.

BRIGHT LIGHT MEDITATION

When we are balanced we are attached to the truth, and not to fear.

- For this meditation, sit in Easy Pose.
- Inhale, and extend your arms straight out to the side, parallel to the ground with your palms facing up.
- As you exhale, bend your elbows and bring your hands up to your shoulders.
- From this position, raise both elbows toward your head, touch your hands behind the back of your neck, lifting the shoulders and the entire spine.
- Lower your elbows as you exhale.
- Continue for three minutes with powerful breathing while you mentally chant the word, "Har," which means God.

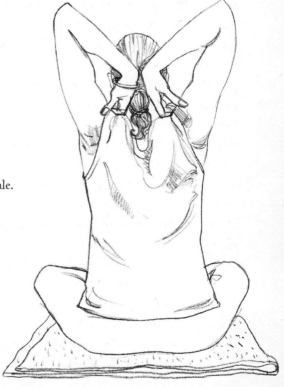

Bright light

. . . AND
BEYOND

*After you have children,
you enter into the
unknown every day.
Be like a river.
Be ever present
and flowing.*

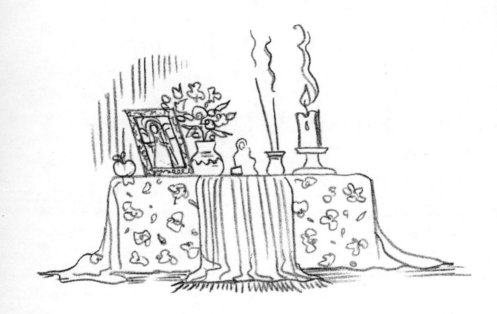

BABY
IN
YOUR ARMS

"We lie,
Noses touching
And I fill my lungs
With your sleeping breath."

—ROHANA VERTCOUTERE

How was your labor? Was it long, short, hard, unbelievable, incredible, had to take drugs, had to have a C-section, everything you dreamed it would be, nothing like you imagined, a nightmare, a spiritual experience? In the end, what really matters and what is the most important thing in your life is holding in your arms a baby who is healthy, complete, whole.

At the turn of the twentieth century, births began to move from homes into hospitals. Women were unconscious because they were totally anesthetized. Since they were knocked out, they couldn't care for their babies, and that began the process of separation, of the baby being moved to a nursery to be cared for by others until the mother could come around. When the birth process is allowed to remain undisturbed, a lot of important things happen in those first few moments and hours after birth. Our bodies are under the effects of natural, opiatelike hormones, which play a role in establishing the conscious bond with our infant. Up until this point, the link has been on a spiritual level, because they were not separate from us. Oxytocin, the love hormone that allows humans to act altruistically, is at the highest peak right after birth. When we look into our baby's eyes and feel his bare skin against our bare skin, we are spiritually forever bonded. A baby is born with big pupils just for this reason, as a call to his mother, "Look into my eyes." I can tell you there is nothing more pure or more profound in the whole world than this. The day Wa was born, the two of us spent the entire day in bed with our eyes on her, and hers on ours. Those hours are stamped on my soul as a time in paradise. I recall the words of my teacher, "In God the child dwells. God is not a church or a temple. God is in the home. The child is born to God. He lives in God, he dwells in God, and he goes in God."

For the next three years, your baby's spirit will be unfolding as a human being. He is learning through all of his senses about trust, intimacy, his identity, feelings of completeness, self-worth, and so much more. Just by holding him, you are giving him what he needs later to be a whole, happy person.

We give birth and then forever and ever will always remember that initiation through what is sometimes referred to as "the ring of fire," that transcendent and awesome experience of feeling the baby move out from your body and enter this earth. Sometimes we can lose sight of the big picture, hold on to our fears and get stuck in the grip of the negative mind. That's how those horror stories you hear while you are pregnant get started. After forty days, mothers return to class to present their children. Sometimes a mother will launch into a story that's really only about herself and what she went through giving birth, forgetting the blessing she holds in her arms. My reply is always the same. Lovingly I say, "Ten toes, ten fingers, beautiful smile. You did the best you could, the doctor or midwife did the best they could. Together you worked very diligently. Now let go, let God. Stare into these eyes. Is there anything in the universe more perfect, more precious, more loving?"

In the hospital, when your baby leaves you, he has no idea where he is being taken when he goes to the nursery. You have been your baby's sole home and experience for nine months. All your baby has done for nine months is hear your heartbeat, feel your body moving, hear your voice and laughter. Your baby's existence was inside feeling you, hearing you, sensing you, seeing you. All of a sudden, your baby is pushed into a strange world, like a fish out of water. He sees you for the first time in your arms, and of course he feels safe and secure, recognizing you, "Yes it is she, the one I know."

But then, boom! What's this? Your baby is taken away by something that smells and seems very different from you and walked down a hall with bright lights that hurts little eyes that have so recently come from the darkness of the womb. I remember a story about a woman who had been in hypnotherapy and in one session relived her own birth. Everything was fine during the birth. She was not troubled or traumatized coming through the birth canal because she remembered it would be this much work. Right after the moment that she remembered the touch of her mother, however, she started to sob uncontrollably. She was remembering being taken down a long, cold hall to the nursery away from her mother! She wept because her body had never forgotten the fear and insecurity of being unceremoniously taken from her mother, who was all she had known and loved for nine months. No one told her where she was going or if she would ever return.

In the late eighties we began to educate mothers about this subject. We told them to explain to their doctors that they did not want to have their baby taken from them except for an emergency, and to please bring the scale into their rooms to weigh the little ones. At first there was such resistance! "Scales don't move, and you don't know how to wash a baby!" We said there was no rush to scrub them up, even much later was fine. The babies just want to be in our arms. We said we would bring our own scales and our own baby tubs, and that is precisely what we did. So today, in most L.A. hospitals, baby can stay with Mom. And Dad—poor Dad! We are working on your being able to sleep with your wife and baby and not on a little cot in the corner of the hospital room. We want the family bed in all hospitals! We need to examine all these practices we have come to accept as part of our experience of what is "normal" infant care.

Remember that a newborn is more intelligent than we are. Think of that when you talk to him—he's smarter and certainly wiser, he just doesn't speak your language yet.

A student gave me an incredible picture of two newborns lying next to each other, one with an arm around the other. The two were twins, and each had been placed in a separate incubator. One was much weaker than the other and not expected to live. A pediatric nurse fought the hospital policy and placed the babies in one incubator. When they were put side by side, the healthier one threw an arm over her sister in an embrace. Almost immediately the weaker baby's heart rate stabilized and her temperature rose to normal. What more evidence do we need? The embrace of those who love us can't be measured. Intelligence is measured in caring and loving; our infants are the masters.

EXERCISE FOR STRONG, LOVING ARMS

This gets your arms strong, and your heart open, ready to receive your baby.

- Begin by stretching your arms out in front of you with your palms firmly pressed together, elbows straight, arms parallel to the floor.
- As you inhale deeply through your nose, open your arms out wide in a large, expansive gesture. Feel the area of your heart open and expand as your lungs fill with air.
- Keep your arms opening and stretching, eventually stretching back as far as they will go, stretching your shoulder blades to touch each other. Really feel the stretch as though your arms were giant wings you are stretching in the bright morning sun. Feel the stretch across your chest, under your arms and your ribs, down the arms and out through the fingertips. Keep your arms parallel to the ground the entire time.
- When your arms are stretched as wide as they can go, begin exhaling through your nose, and bring your arms back to the original position, ending with your palms pressed together once again.
- Do this twenty-six times with your eyes closed and rolled up to your Third Eye point.

- Remember to inhale and exhale powerfully, silently reciting "Sat" on the inhale and "Nam" on the exhale.
- Move at a moderate pace. Your arms and heart will be so ready to receive the one. This is good for Dad to do also.

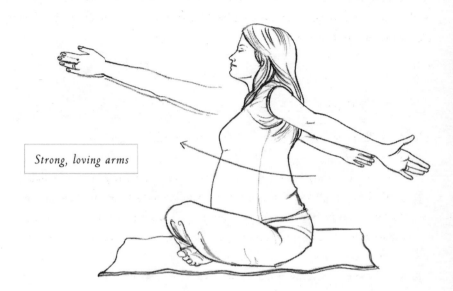

Strong, loving arms

ADVICE AND OPTIONS ON NURSING YOUR BABY

The power of mother's milk. Your milk is your blood turned into life-sustaining food for your baby. According to the ancient texts, your blood is your personality, as in "she is hot-blooded," "he is cold-blooded." The power of mother's milk from this perspective is in putting your personality in the nourishment you give your child. It is your life force, your essential energy, that you give. That is why it is so important to nurse if it is possible for you to do so.

There are occasionally physical reasons why it is not possible to nurse, but sometimes, such as in the case of not enough milk, those challenges can usually be solved. Resting, relaxing, and sleeping probably help the most, because you must support your body in its need to harness the tremendous energy it takes to create milk. (There is a powerful tea called "Mother's Milk" made by Traditional Medicinals, which is great for milk production.)

Above all, *don't give up!* Try every possibility and use that patience you learned in pregnancy. In this country there are wonderful resources like La Leche League that can help. Hospitals often have a lactation consultant who can offer hands-on help.

Call friends who are nursing and talk with them about what they've learned. If you have a doula for after the birth helping in the house, she can be a great resource as well. When we women put our heads together, an answer can always be found. In Los Angeles, we have a wonderful resource called the Pump Station, wonderful women who care for breast-feeding mothers. (You can call from anywhere in the country, see "Inspired Resources," page 229.)

Before you go into labor, have a phone number for a lactation consultant by the side of your bed. The first ten days are often the most challenging. *Don't give up.* As we say in Kundalini yoga, Keep up! Sometimes it seems that the baby doesn't want the breast, but every baby wants to nurse. Have faith that he will get the knack. It could come down to simply shifting his position in your arms. If you don't get it easily, don't beat yourself up, get help. It's okay not to know. Most of us need help—I sure did.

Take the time to nurse, because you will be giving your child the most important gift you can for his immune system, nervous system, skeletal system, brain, every part of him. It's recently been discovered that children who breast-feed may grow up to be smarter adults. A recent study published in the *Journal of the American Medical Association* concluded that adults who were breast-fed from seven to nine months had higher IQs than those who were breast-fed for less than two weeks. Mother's milk contains a polyunsaturated acid that researchers think protects or even stimulates our central nervous system. Another vital element is more difficult to measure, and is priceless: the time and attention you give as you nurse your baby at your breast. That alone raises IQ. Another study from the journal *Pediatrics* found that breast-feeding may actually protect infants from pain. In this study, crying and grimacing decreased 91 percent in infants having their blood drawn while at their mother's breast. Taste, suckling, and skin-to-skin contact are known to relieve pain in animals, but this was the first study to say the benefits likely extends to humans.

And this is all accomplished through your milk. See how amazing you are, Mom? A child can grow round and happy for an entire year on your milk alone. That's how great you are.

Just make sure you continue to eat as well as you did while you were pregnant—remember, unprocessed foods, not prepackaged, and as full of *prana* as possible. Frozen food and canned foods are the last choice. Remember, alive, fresh and organic, as best you can. What goes in your mouth creates your blood, and your blood creates your milk. Babies are at the top of the food chain—they eat from you, so give them a delicious feast of healthy milk. The ancients knew that certain foods would bring in milk and help tone the uterus, like ginger curry, tapioca pudding made with milk or soy, sautéed almonds, mung beans and rice, and Yogi Tea with milk or soy. If your milk supply runs dry, it usually is telling you you're running around too much, tired, and perhaps not eating well. It takes a lot of energy to produce milk. Sleep, relax, sleep, and drink lots of the tea Mother's Milk by Traditional Medicinals. Milk almost always comes back plentifully.

When you nurse, nurse. Don't do five million other things at the same time. It would be like someone coming to your house for a dinner party and reading a book or talking on the phone the entire time. How rude would that be? Yet, do we do this exact thing when we nurse? A good meal comes from the company you are with, the conversation, eye contact, and love shared!

What if you just cannot nurse because you have had surgery that cut through your milk ducts, or some other medical reason? Research to find the very best mother's milk substitute you can find. *Mothering* magazine's on-line site is a great resources (see "Inspired Resources," page 229). When I was a child, there was a contraption for infants that balanced a bottle on a baby's chest. The idea was to not have to hold your infant as you fed her. She ate alone, by herself. I wonder what that generation of babies who ate that way are doing now. Eating by themselves alone, still? Even if you cannot nurse, hold your baby in the same position as if you were nursing when you give the bottle.

When my daughter was an infant there were no breast pumps, at least that I knew about, so that wasn't a choice. Today mothers freeze their milk so when they go back to their jobs they can have someone give the milk by bottle. If you must, you must, but if you absolutely do not have to, why do it? Nothing in the universe will ever take the place of your very own breast and nipple—nothing ever! I never had to give my daughter a bottle. When she did begin to eat food and drink, I gave her a sippy cup at five months, but before that I put water on a little spoon and she took it easily.

Thankfully, our culture is becoming more aware of this, and more support for breast-feeding can be found. I received the following letter from Blair, a longtime student and mother of two. I found it so encouraging I wanted to share it with you. She writes:

Due to some mishaps while delivering Lily last year, I had some apprehension about the maternity staff at the hospital. I found myself one day asking to see a woman named Nancy, head of maternity for the hospital. Her assistant insisted I meet Nancy for lunch. Nancy greeted me and introduced me to the head nurse. There was a beautiful lunch set up in a conference room just for the three of us. They asked me to relay my concerns and requests. They said since the last time I had given birth the maternity ward had been completely transformed. It is totally pro-breast-feeding with lactation help around the clock and support groups for breast-feeding. Also, everything with baby is done in our room. Their goal is for the baby never to have to go to the nursery. I had a lot of fuzzy information cleared up on the eyedrop and the Vitamin K shot they give newborns, and, now with clarity, have made my decision on those issues. I also was introduced to the head lactation consultant. I was able to share the things we talked about in our yoga class; they were all very open about it. The hospital is awaiting their "Baby Friendly Status"— apparently only 19 hospitals in the country have this. It's a worldwide movement to promote breast-feeding by the hospitals.

They all gave me their cards and said, "We want to know when you arrive. . . ."

I never would have done this prior to yoga and meditation. The whole experience was empowering. For a change, I trusted and followed my intuition to take care of myself and baby. By some miracle, I was not confrontational, just mildly assertive, so I was met with a very warm response. Now I feel so, so covered on the spiritual AND the medical end. But of course: God is everything, after all. We just have to look for him, even in unlikely places. . . .

Much love,

Blair (and Lily, Dante and Baby Liam)

ULTIMATE EXERCISE FOR BETTER NURSING

Be confident that you have all you need to produce complete nourishment for your child. Plan on being rather dreamy for the first year of your child's life, if only because the energy to produce milk is so internal and miraculous. Slow down and live as simply as possible with your new family to give your child the security she needs.

Better nursing

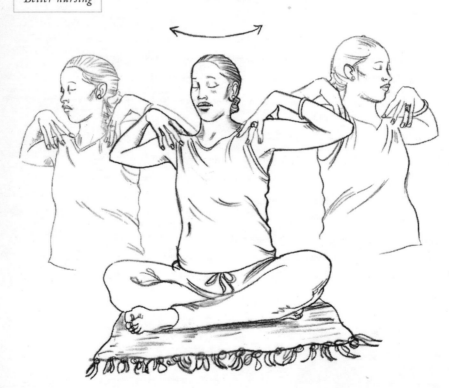

- Sit in Easy Pose on the floor.
- Grasp your shoulders with your fingers in front, thumbs in the back.
- Close your eyes.
- Inhale through your nose and twist to the left, exhale through your nose and twist to the right.
- Inhale the sound "Sat" silently as you turn to the left, and exhale "Nam" silently as you turn to the right.
- Do this for three minutes. This opens your heart center, improves circulation, and purifies the blood that makes milk.

INCLUDING YOUR COMMUNITY: FORTY-DAY CELEBRATION

L ooking at babies is like looking at God. That's why everybody wants to be around them—they all want to be in the presence of God! As proud as you are, this is when you and the baby need to be quiet and private during this delicate time right after the baby has come.

In our families, as given to us from the ancient teachings, we observe forty days of sacred privacy and quiet for the mother and baby. It is a time of rest, rejuvenation, and bonding for Mom, Baby, Dad, and your other children. In this time, the intimacy of the magnetic field between the mother and child is confirmed, and the deepest core values of security are transmitted. This is called molding. Babies need more time, because they are not finished "baking" yet. Bring them into the world slowly, one day for each of the forty weeks (or so) they grew in your womb. This also gives the baby's immune system time to develop before being exposed to bacteria and viruses from the outside world.

These forty days can be an incredible time in your family's life. It's like watching a rose open and open—*don't lose this magic, because it doesn't come around again.*

Forty days, historically, has been a significant time period for many world faiths. In the Old Testament, it rained for forty days and forty nights, and it took Noah forty days to build the Ark; the Christians observe forty days of Lent. Jesus meditated in the desert for forty days. There are forty days of Ramadan in the Muslim faith. Forty-day cycles are very important to my faith as well. It is also significant that our physical body renews all the cells in our bloodstream every forty days. Forty days is a number representing completion.

During these days, you might want to choose those certain foods from the previous chapter that bring in milk and help heal the uterus. Ideally someone else needs to prepare your meals, because during this time a mother needs to do as little as possible. Food preparation, cleaning, and laundry need to be put in the care of someone—a helper, a family member, or a close friend. We say that it's good to sleep when the baby sleeps, because otherwise it can take up to two and a half years to regain your full strength rather than a mere forty days.

If you have friends and relatives you feel nurtured by, have them help you with errands, shopping, whatever needs to get done. If friends ask, "What can I do to help?" never reply, "Nothing." One student has a very close friend who lives in another state. These two women have been best friends since they were children, practically all their lives. Both times the friend out of state has given birth, our student gives her the best possible baby present: She takes a flight out to spend ten days with her best friend, cooking and cleaning, caring for the older child, and handling phone calls so that the family can be together and her friend can rest and restore herself. It's time she happily gives as an expression of her deep love for her friend, and she will likely receive the same when it's her turn to have a child! If you have other children and you have friends who are good with kids, have them take the kids to the park or to a playground for some fun. It is wonderful to be able to hire an after-birth doula, if that is at all possible. It's ideal if you can stay within nine feet of your baby for these days, to solidify the aura, the link of energy, between the two of you. It will last a lifetime.

Some of us might fear surrendering to this process, afraid we will lose our independence and identity as a person by living so completely as a mother. Let me assure you that these forty days are beautiful, necessary, and a vital phase for the baby's development of security in themselves, God and the innate knowingness of how to love and be loved that will be with them for the rest of their lives. How they find their mate, marry, and have families is very much influenced by the experience of these forty days. This time is important for your own healing, and for your family to honor the transition of another member back to earth. But this golden time will not last forever. Still, for now, considerations and worries about finances, work, or the opinions of others need to fade into the background. You never will have this time again, and it goes by so quickly.

Maria is a newspaper reporter who only recently gave birth to her second child, a baby boy named Cruz. Her daughter is in preschool. Maria has just turned thirty-nine, and she and her husband have decided not to try for any more children. She told me: "This time with Cruz is so special. I realize I will never again have a baby nurse, or hear his coos. I didn't realize until he came along just how much I had taken for granted with the birth of my daughter. I feel like I don't want to miss anything now!" She has arranged to file her stories for the newspaper by computer and work from home a couple days a week. "I don't want to lose this time with my babies."

The forty days ends with a celebration of community. We have a "coming out" celebration in our homes or temples. Mama and baby are presented to the world with singing and dancing, poetry, food, and flowers. Everyone brings gifts for the baby, just as in the celebration at one hundred and twenty days all the gifts are for Mom.

I encourage you to take any part, or all, of our tradition and make it your own celebration for your family, friends, and community. I recently ran into Julie, a former student from one of the first prenatal classes I ever taught seven years ago who was rediscovering her yoga practice. Of course we caught up on each other's lives, and she happened to mention that one of the things she still treasures is the forty-day rest and celebration.

"It just resonated with me. So many of the teachings just felt like the right thing. Truth is truth. I knew my rabbi agreed. There wasn't anything in the Kundalini practice that went against my teachings. All good comes down to the same thing in the end, I believe," Julie told me. "With my son, a doctor's checkup was the only time we went out. People thought I was nuts, my Jewish friends were like, 'Oh great, here we go with the New Age stuff,' but I didn't care. I am a person who has dealt with a lot of anxiety in my life, and I felt very connected to my child in that time. It was a general feeling of well-being."

For the birth of her second child, the process was a little different because she had to care for her son at the same time. "My daughter stayed home for forty days, but I had a little more running around to do. Still, I didn't go out of my way to go do things," Julie confided. "I knew how important the time was, because I will never forget the first time my son and I went down the street for a walk. He covered his tiny ears with his little hands to block out the street sounds we just take for granted. At that moment, I said a prayer of thanks that I was able to introduce him to it slowly."

We have twin sisters who have each come to prenatal classes three different times for their three separate children. Recently one of the sisters returned yet again, and I was so happy to see her. They both were born and raised in L.A. and are very close to their whole family. Their babies are all born in their parents' home. After the births of their children, the twins and their husbands live at the parents' house and the parents take care of everyone during the forty days. It's a beautiful setup, and unique—so many of us in L.A. are originally from other parts of the country or the globe and have family scattered all over. I just love old-fashioned arrangements that work!

MEDITATION FOR
CONNECTING TO FAMILY

- Breathe in and out deeply through your nose a few times.
- Then scrunch your shoulders up tightly to your ears, then relax and lower your shoulders. Do this at least five times.

- Next, close your eyes and roll your head around, first to the right, then to the left, inhaling and exhaling deeply through your nose.
- Bring your head up and roll your eyes up to your Third Eye point. Start singing the sound "Ong," curling your tongue and pressing the back of the tongue against the back of the throat firmly. Do this for three to seven minutes.
- It will sound as if you are singing "Onnnng" through your nose. Feel how good this sound feels running through you. "Ong" means Infinity in its most creative form. . . . Hey, that sounds a lot like you right now!

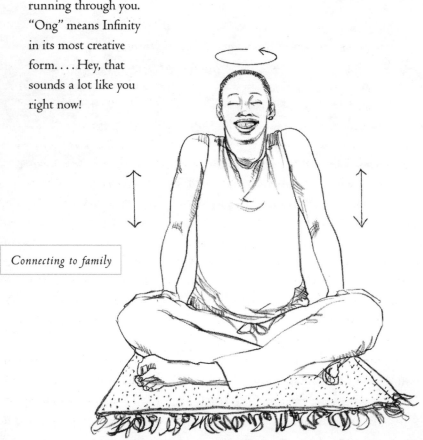

Connecting to family

ESTABLISHING
NEW ROLES
AND TRADITIONS

"It doesn't take
centuries. It takes
moments, and
those are the
happiest moments."

— YOGI BHAJAN

Let me tell you a little story about our dear student Rebecca, who came back to Los Angeles after leaving her conservative Jewish family here to be married in New York. She was very young, in her early twenties. She began coming to class early in her pregnancy, and then she started researching some of the topics I bring up in class—and have brought to you in this book. She decided to have a home birth. She also decided, based on her research, that there was no proof of circumcision being a medical necessity. The American Medical Association and the American Pediatric Association are no longer endorsing this procedure, insurance companies are no longer paying for it, and in fact a group of pediatricians are trying to make it illegal, calling it child mutilation without their consent.

Circumcision is one ancient ritual that has been practiced throughout the world. For Jews and Muslims, it has been a religious ritual, while in other countries like Africa it is one of the rites for puberty. The United States is the only country that practices routine circumcision for nonreligious reasons. We have translated the structures from ancient history into this modern society of ours. Where people once looked to a priest, it seems we look to a doctor; where people long ago went to a temple, we go to a hospital. Pharmaceuticals seem to be the sacraments of today.

Even though it was practiced in their religion, Rebecca and her husband agreed it was *more* important *not* to circumcise their son.

When her parents found out her plans, at first they didn't take her seriously. "You're too young to know what you're talking about," they told her. But she stuck to her guns, and her husband supported her. Then her parents got angry. "If you do this, you will be cut out of your inheritance and we will disown you and our grand-child," they vowed. Even after the baby was born, her mother was still raging at her.

Finally, Rebecca knew she needed to take a stand. "I will not accept you addressing me with this kind of disrespect," she told her mother, "and I will not let you make decisions for my family." Then, she did a very difficult thing for a daughter who loved and honored her parents: She forbade them to the house until they were willing to respect her as the matriarch of her own family. Rebecca knew she had to protect her son and her husband from the negative, stressful environment arguing and raised voices creates.

It was challenging, and there were a lot of tears on both sides. Since Rebecca took that stand, her parents realized she was serious, and, ultimately, that she had the strength of her convictions, an important quality for all of us! Eventually, her parents came around to accept her commitment. In fact, Rebecca's mother has had a complete change of heart. She now says, "I don't see how anyone could circumcise their sons!"

You are the ultimate authority for your child's welfare, period. No matter how helpful grandparents and extended family can be, "the buck stops with you," as the saying goes. Traditions can be important for families and for cultural unity. Please consider, for a moment, that a soul is born complete, that the foreskin of a man's penis is not an abnormality. The foreskin protects the glans of a man's penis throughout his life, and it's now known that good personal hygiene provides all the protection against infection, which makes the idea of routine circumcision obsolete. I think it is wonderful and important to carry out traditions, but I suggest having the ceremony without the actual cutting and pain you inflict upon your son. Be creative! There are many ways to celebrate the covenant of God and your son. There are ways to honor your family and still respect your infant son. I always think about this quote from the book, *The Sayings of Jesus*: "If circumcision were useful, we would be born without foreskins."

Now that you are a mother, recast your own self-image as the "child" of your parents to being a parent in your own right. Do it with grace, with dignity, and with prayer. Set the parameters early about what you want for your own family, and they will respect you. If they don't, reevaluate their role in your life. If they don't respect you now, when will they? When you stand up and assume your role as the parent, you might be surprised at how that frees them and allows them to accept their position as grandparents.

Grandparents have a job: to spoil their grandkids with love and attention. They did the work of raising you, so now they can enjoy their grandchildren without the pressure of ultimate responsibility. Let them be available to offer wisdom to both you and your children.

SONG OF GRATITUDE AND LOVE

This is the song we sing at the child's birth as a welcoming song into the world. At the end of all our classes we sing it:

> *May the long time sun shine upon you*
> *All love surround you*
> *And the pure light within you*
> *Guide your way on*

Say it to all those people in your life, for your children's grandparents, your parents, because they gave you your life. Leave all judgments behind. They gave you life, and if you cannot bless them for anything else, bless them for that, because you would not have this experience of being a parent without the one egg and the one sperm that came together. You would not be you without them, amazing you! In your most challenging moments, parents will respect this prayer. In fact, put it on your fridge, on your answering machine, birth announcements, wherever you like. It brings trust and love and sunshine. We never tire of it!

THE FAMILY
BED

Many other cultures look on our need to have a nursery or a baby's room with the perfect bassinet, changing table, mobile, and so on, in amazement. Anthropologists say that in most cultures in the world, the baby and children share the bed with the parents. The number who strive for the pattern we have, the baby down the hall in the nursery, is exactly . . . zero.

Your baby does not need or want a fancy crib or nursery, only your physical closeness. Just as a joey only needs its kangaroo mother's pouch, so too will your baby be nurtured by closeness to you. A baby's needs can't be met by going to a toy store or having the most fancy stroller in town. Just remember the two Ts: Touch and Tenderness. My teacher once said that "a child needs the psyche to grow in the realm of courage. What can counseling do when insecurity has gone into the very genes of the child, and he is alone?" In some countries, in fact, they would never put a child in a stroller to be pushed in front of his mom. Where is the protection? Babies in most countries go on Mom or behind her!

Sleep with your baby and don't get so carried away with schedules. When a baby cries, she usually is telling you: I am hungry, I am tired, I need to have my diaper changed, I want to be held. It's a simple equation: How does she know she's hungry? Her stomach growls and wakes her up! She really doesn't want to wake you up to come down the hall to feed her, but her tummy won't stop growling till she does. How much better if she is only right there by your side in bed. A baby will create her own schedule, and it will be a very fine schedule for her. It will be her schedule and as unique and magical as she is.

You might have heard about the concept of patterning your baby's sleep periods so you can get her to sleep through the night. I see mothers come into class, and they are so eager to tell us that they got their baby to sleep through the night. "I'm so pleased!" they say. What's to be proud of there? Is it a competition? Some mothers are then led to think there is something wrong with them, because they can't get their child to sleep through the night.

In so many other places in the world, Mom and Dad sleep with their baby in the bed. When she nurses, she nurses, when she wakes, she wakes. But we are so methodical here. We read these books that offer a "plan," like letting a child cry and cry. Mothers come to me very upset, saying, "I am trying to get my baby to sleep through the night, but I can't let him cry." Well, don't. Pick him up and nurse him!

So much information new moms receive is about trying to get your child to "fit" into your life. What you must do, and you will enjoy doing, is creating a new life for all of you—baby, Mom, and Dad. In a year, your baby will probably be talking, and walking away from you a little farther and farther for the rest of his or her life. And that's what we want them to do—be strong and independent beings. *The time with your baby during pregnancy and the first year will never come around again.* Please do not try to make this time regular or ordinary. Please do not try to figure it out. What I am saying is, you need a life less complicated. Simplify, simplify, simplify. Surrender, surrender, surrender. Live each precious moment.

When you were a kid, what was the first thing you wanted to do when you got up? Jump in your parents' bed, no doubt. It's natural in a healthy family for children to want to be close. By the same token, it's fine for children to have their own rooms as they grow older, too, so they can have space when they need their own private time, but it's not a necessity.

In the sixties, I hitchhiked by myself all through Mexico—thankfully I am still alive to tell the tale. I was south of Oaxaca, and I wanted so much to live like a native Indian. Honestly, I didn't have a clue about the difference in tribes and cultures among the indigenous people, I just knew I didn't want to be living an ordinary American life, so I sought out native people. They thought I was very odd—what was I doing, this crazy girl, trying to look like them? But they opened their huts to me, and I learned a lot. One thing that struck me was how they were with their children. For one, the parents were always carrying them. It was a practical arrangement: They had to work so they carried their children. This bond wasn't some mystical, woo-woo thing, it was daily life. When the babies were not on their mama's body, they were above the family, looking down. They used Coca-Cola crates as baskets strung by rope high above the floor of their huts to keep the babies safe from bugs and animals. The lovely thing I always noticed was that throughout the day the family would go by and gently push the side of the crate so the bassinet was always rocking back and forth, and the baby got to watch the comings and goings from a ringside seat.

After Wa was born, someone gave me a one-person soft woven hammock. One day I just hoisted it above the kitchen table, I put a sheepskin in there, and laid her in it. She would look down, look up, like a little bird in a nest. Whoever was near the hammock would gently push it so she was constantly swaying back and forth. She loved to "hang out" in it.

If you go into one of these big baby stores, you walk away thinking you have to have the deluxe super baby buggy, fancy changing table, the mobile for above the crib, and a digital bottle warmer to be a good parent. Not really. You don't have to have anything special to be a great parent except your arms. Can't afford a changing table? Change your baby on the bed! It's so logical when you remove yourself from all that marketing aimed at you and tune in to your heart and your baby's. What does this little soul need? Not all babies, just this baby. Tune in to your intuition and your all-knowingness, to your self-knowledge and who you are. You chose your baby and your baby chose you. It is a glorious contract.

When Wa was born, she never slept away from me and her Papa. It was so wonderful, because even if Papa hadn't had the chance to spend that much time with her that day because he was away at work, it gave him a way to be part of the experience. At night you travel on the same dreams together. Imagine waking up in the morning and gazing into each other's eyes, just you, your partner, and your baby, or just watching them sleep next to you, wrapped in their scent, listening to them breathe softly in and out. *There is nothing in the world like it.*

If you want to get cozy with your partner, simply snuggle your baby next to your back so you can snuggle with your partner. What if you want to make love? Leave the baby to snooze in the bed and the two of you go to another room or find other creative places in your house. Now's the time for some imagination—and it can be really fun.

Mothers and dads wonder if they will have trouble sleeping. Some nights, Dad ends up on the couch, or you end up in another room feeding the baby. It's often musical beds. I would get up in the morning and wonder, Did Wa wake up last night? Because it all turns into a dream. When Wa started rolling over at night, we put the mattress on the floor so she wouldn't have anywhere to fall and stored the bed frame in the garage for a while. When she started crawling, we child-proofed the room so she could go anywhere off the bed and be perfectly safe. I would wake up to see her in a corner on the other side of the room, fast asleep. To this day she is very flexible in her physical body and mind. She can still sleep anywhere and is spontaneous in almost any situation.

After you have children, you enter into the unknown every day. Do what you can do when you can do it, because children are always the unpredictable element. Don't try to figure everything out, because as soon as you do, they are on to something else. Be like a river. Be ever present and flowing.

I am writing this at a painful time in history after the September 11, 2001, tragedy in New York, Washington, and Pennsylvania where terrorists took the lives of thousands of people, and the world faces much hardship. Let us hold each other, let families sleep together, and then our nation will be together. Peace and solidarity begin at home. When my teacher came to America from India in 1969, he, in his hard-to-understand, heavily accented English, would often use the word "cozy." We thought it was a corny word, but more and more over time I have come to appreciate and feel the depth of this simple four-letter word. Cozy fills you up with good feelings. Like a cat and her kittens, be cozy in your family bed. Sweet dreams!

FACING THE CHALLENGE OF TOMORROW TOGETHER

- With your partner, come sitting on the floor, sitting on your heels if possible. If you cannot do this sit in Easy Pose.
- Have your knees touching your partner's and clasp hands. Now, both of you lean back as far as is comfortable.
- Shut your eyes and inhale the sound "Sat," exhale the sound "Nam" through your mouth with a long, even breath so the sound becomes "Naaaaaaam."
- Do this for three minutes, then come back to center. Don't forget to kiss each other for the grand finale!

Facing the challenge of tomorrow

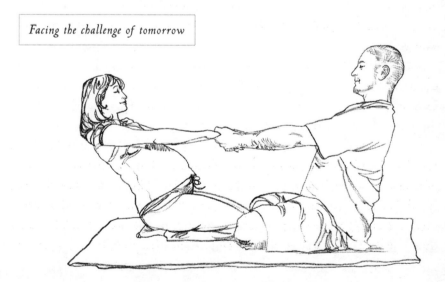

TIME ENOUGH:
THE TRANSITION
OF THE FAMILY

*"Life can never be
'the way it used to be.'
Evolution doesn't
go backwards."*

—JACOB LIBERMAN,
*WISDOM FROM AN
EMPTY MIND*

People are always surprised at the joyful ruckus that erupts from the postpartum yoga classes—there's a lot of cooing and crying, laughing and talking that goes on as infants to toddlers interact with their mommies doing yoga. While pregnancy is a kind of dream time, full of wonder and wishes for the future, life with baby throws you, full-tilt, into *real* time. There are dirty diapers, sleepless nights, a lot of juggling and a lot more noise! And here is where you start to see the true, everlasting joy of having a family: Once the baby has arrived, the paradox hits you that life is uncomfortable and chaotic and more astounding, more amazing, than you ever dreamed it could be.

With all the hustle and bustle of just making it through the day, it's sometimes easy to forget that a huge and important transition is taking place. You have gone from wondering about nursing to bringing milk in, from imagining and dreaming what your baby will look like to actually caring for the little soul in your arms. Every day a metamorphosis is occurring: You wake up and there is a more fully realized soul next to you, changing as if before your eyes. The speed that we see children grow is amazing, and the experiences you and your family share now change you all forever. Having an awareness of this alone can help smooth the challenges of this transition time.

Besides having a baby, you are now a family, or a bigger family! With this new being in the house, you'll be reinspired by the new and deeper connection to your partner.

If you have other children they will be wondering how they fit into this new arrangement. So many times I have women come to my classes for their second pregnancy who are concerned. "How is this going to work? *How am I going to have time for everything?*" they ask. One woman had a three-year-old, and was worried over stories she heard that young children sometimes regress back to diapers and infant behavior when the new soul arrives. On occasion this can happen, but certainly not as often as the urban wives' tales would have you believe. We all hear stories but it's only the bad ones that "stick on the page." With the knowingness that your child will indeed transition into the role of big brother or big sister, use these two tools to help it along: *Allow and include.*

Allow your other children to go through the transition by giving love and understanding at every turn, not judgment and punishment. Get them talking and expressing how they feel. Include them in this new miracle. If you have a family bed, get them right in there with you, perhaps next to Papa. Allow them to "help" you if they like, and when the new baby is sleeping take time with big brother or big sister. Reading a story and then some conversation just with them alone will go a long way in letting them know their place in your heart is unchanged. Children are unconditional in their love for you. What you say means the world to them. Explain why you had to take the attention off them for a while to help usher their baby sister or brother into the world. Give your children respect; they are truly wise. Everything will work itself out a day at a time . . . a few days at a time! Find a way where just you and the baby and big brother or sister can go out together, even to the store or the park for an hour.

Sometimes I hear mothers say, "I love my child so much, I can't imagine loving more. Where will the love come from for the new child on the way?" That is one of the true blessings of having children; they give you a direct experience of the bounty of the world. The truth is there is a bountifulness in love. It expands exponentially the minute you give to another. The fear that there isn't enough is just a delusion of scarcity. Not only is there enough love for your new child, there is more love for your partner than you ever imagined, and the love you can create for your children is beyond measure. Love creates love. You don't have to believe it. It's a fact. It just is.

"THERE'S LOVE ENOUGH FOR EVERYTHING" EXERCISE

This exercise stimulates the heart chakra, reminding us of the limitlessness of love:

- Sit on your heels or in Easy Pose with a straight spine, your hands at the center of your chest in Prayer Pose.
- Focus your eyes at the tip of your nose.
- Begin to extend your arms fully out to your sides as if you are pressing against two walls, then return to the starting position.
- As you move your arms, repeat the sound "Hummmmmm" out loud, with your lips coming together as if to create a gentle buzzing, like the sound of a bee. "Hum" is the sound that opens the heart. Continue for three to seven minutes.

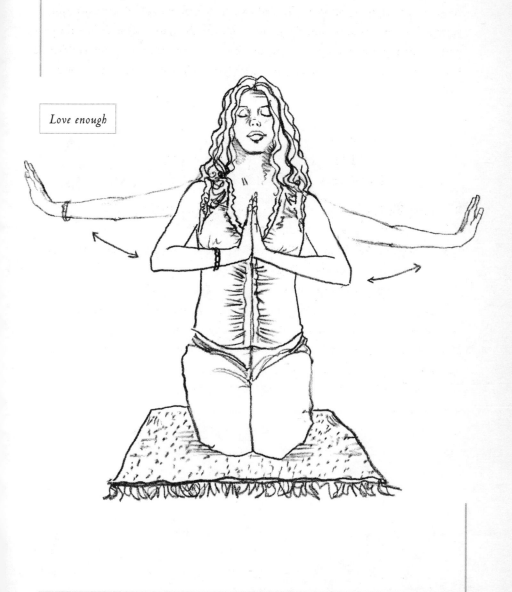

Love enough

THE INFINITE
HORIZON OF A
MOTHER'S LOVE

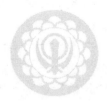

Being a great and happy parent is a big job and an honorable one. It is a chance to do your part in giving to the world. Right now, you might be up to your ears in diapers, not have had time to take a shower, be unable to find the cordless phone, and you read these words and think, "What? I have to save the world, too? It's too much!" But it's true. The only way this planet will fulfill its destiny toward enlightenment, when love and brotherhood will reign, is if each of us, within ourselves and in our homes, creates a space for love to grow.

We had a beautiful student at our center some years ago. She went to full term with a complicated pregnancy, but then had a son with physical problems. This happens so rarely. After eighteen years of teaching pregnant women, I can count on one hand the number whose babies have not come happy and healthy. This little fellow had a different destiny than many, and after a short time, he passed.

The mother grieved hard, and then she put that grief to work. She discovered there was a huge need in the Los Angeles area for a playground accessible to children with disabilities. And so she began raising money by coordinating benefits and auctions. She was able to get a lot of press attention, and her hard work, and that of many others who joined her mission, resulted in a beautiful children's park. All the equipment is accessible to children with disabilities, although all children are welcomed to join the fun.

Now she is working on getting a second park up and running. Let us learn from her: She took that singular love for her one baby and extended it out to all children. What you give, you receive, and now, I am happy to say, she has a birthed a second child, a very healthy and happy baby girl.

Can we love not just our own child, but love their playmates down the street with a great amount of care, and also ferocity? Can we love the children half a world away who speak a different language, who worship in a different way the same God who is in us all? We have an unending capacity for love. Love builds on love; the more, the more. That your children may see you and watch you in that infinite, universal love is one of the greatest gifts you can give them.

MOTHER POWER MEDITATION

This meditation is called "Mother Power":

- Sit with a straight spine in Easy Pose with your hands at your knees in *gyan mudra*, pressing your index finger to your thumb.
- Chant the sound "Maaaaa" eight times per breath for three to seven minutes.
- Then, sit quietly and see light expanding throughout your heart.

FINAL
THOUGHTS:
A NEW WORLD

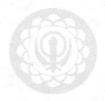

*"Each of you who studies these ancient teachings and
puts them into practice in your life is a pioneer
of the new age. You are the historical crest of hope
and development that will usher in
a new level of consciousness and civilization.
Each of your efforts gives birth to the Aquarian Age."*

—YOGI BHAJAN

Angels arrive without wings, so we have to see them for their smiles. In these past years of teaching mothers and fathers and babies, I have seen nothing but angels in all forms, shapes, and colors. During a trip to Costa Rica, where I taught a yoga retreat, I encountered a little girl who stands out in my mind. She and her mother had come from Boston to be with us for the week.

The mother had begun a yoga and meditation practice while pregnant and never stopped. Her little girl was only seven years old, but she asked to get up at 4 A.M. with us in order to come to *sadhana* and morning yoga each day. In her yoga, she was as steady and focused as an adult—more than some! She had been doing yoga before she was even born in the security of her mother's belly. She was the kind of girl who even at her young age wrote poems in her journal, and spoke with a voice as clear and bright as a bell. One day we all went on a field trip through the Costa Rican jungle to see amazing waterfalls. I saw her off to one side of the group. When I looked, what did she have but Monarch butterflies all around her! She was watching one delicately flutter in her palm, not holding it, just providing it a space to be. The picture was so beautiful it brings tears to my eyes even as I recall it.

Is hers the face of what is possible when mothers and fathers commit themselves to an awakened life? I think so.

Children born now are on the vanguard of the Age of Aquarius. Sometimes called "indigo babies" for the deep blue of the aura they are said to radiate, these children are more aware and present an evolution in spiritual consciousness. In other words, the Age of Aquarius children have a higher frequency of intelligence. We are not going to be able to get anything by them, so now is the time to begin to clear our minds. Let our mission as parents be to help them reach their potential greatness. In that greatness is born a consciousness that will heal the world through light and unconditional love.

In this Aquarian Age we are going into, the ethos will be "I know, therefore I believe." How will you know? From the very core of your being. It has been decreed that the time to *search* for God is over; now is the time to know God in ourselves. "The time has come for self-value," my teacher has said. This shift is a radical difference in perspective from the Piscean Age mankind has been under for the past two thousand years. In this time we have tended to say, "If the priest/rabbi/elder/doctor said so, then I believe." The transition between the Piscean Age and the new Age of Aquarius extends from 1991 to 2012, a twenty-one-year period of passage. This is a time for each one of us to realize and embrace the truth of who we are.

Science is just beginning to catch up. After examining fifteen thousand babies, researchers in China have suggested brain structures may be altering. This relates to something Yogi Bhajan predicted in 1992, that we would witness an evolution in the consciousness of children. Let us look to our children as our teachers; we must continually strive to become more aware and have greater mastery of ourselves, if only to keep up with the glorious children coming through to us now.

I pray the previous pages have given you a window into possibilities for pregnancy and parenting you might not have known about or considered. Because of the time we find ourselves in, it's more important than ever to question the ways and methods we are using to bring children into, and raise them in, this world. The French researcher Michel Odent I referenced in this book has posed the question, "For humans, we must always introduce the question of civilization: What is the future of a civilization born under drugs and anesthesia?" Among us, there is a belief that in five generations the Earth will become pure; in fact that is the meaning of the Khalsa, "pure ones." We don't need more humans on the planet—we need more excellent humans, loving, secure humans to lead us out of the confusion of present times into an age of enlightenment where the highest human quality will be compassion, an open heart.

I have said this before, but it bears repeating: You may think you are just having a baby, but in reality you have the chance to do nothing short of save the world. Take his Holiness the Dalai Lama, for instance. Look at what the contribution of just one little man can do! Understand the incredible opportunity to change the world by changing your consciousness, and the consciousness of your family.

Look at the past, at how many of us didn't want to grow up because we saw our parents' generation and said, "Forget it, I'm not going to be that unhappy, that trapped, that caught up in unpleasantness."

You have a tremendous opportunity right now to become the people who are the shining examples of adulthood, so that your children look to you and say, "My parents are great examples to follow!" The tools provided in this book can be one of your most valuable assets in accomplishing this. I encourage you with all my heart to continue to incorporate Kundalini yoga and meditation in your daily routine. I especially encourage you to take a yoga class of any kind. The benefits of the group energy will only multiply the effect of the work. The greatest gift you can give your child, and every child, is becoming a grateful, graceful, conscious adult who walks mindfully in the world. May amazing grace guide your way on.

MEDITATION FOR
CREATING A BEAUTIFUL WORLD

This powerful meditation helps to bring healing and peace to our planet, and is meant to be done for forty days.

- Sit tall with a straight spine, pulling your chin slightly in, chest out, shoulders relaxed.
- Place the hands in Prayer Pose at the center of your chest, pressing your palms firmly together.
- Roll your eyes up to your Third Eye point and imagine you are sitting atop a tall mountain overlooking all of humanity, and sending waves of peace over the entire globe.
- The mantra, "Ra Ma Da Sa Sa Say So Hung," is a very powerful sound current and has immediate effects to bring healing to yourself and others. The sounds translate as:

Ra = Sun
Ma = Moon
Da = Earth
Sa = Infinity
Say = Totality of experience
So Hung = I am Thou

"Ra Ma Da Sa" melody bar

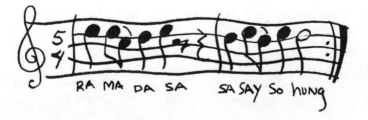

- Chant out loud for twelve minutes, chant in a whisper for five minutes, and be silent for one minute. End by inhaling deeply, and as you exhale sit for a little bit and give this prayer to those who need it.

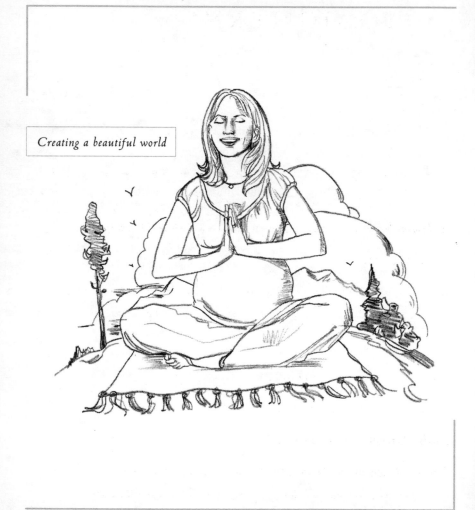

Creating a beautiful world

GLOSSARY
OF
YOGIC TERMS

Ambrosial hours: Early morning, about two hours before the sun rises.

Asana: Yogic posture.

Chakra: Spinning vortexes of energy throughout your body, each radiating a particular energy that is important for your health, happiness, and well-being.

Dharma: Life path.

Guru: That which brings you from darkness into light.

Karma: Cosmic law of cause and effect.

Khalsa: Literally means "pure one."

Kriya: Literally means "a completed action"; yoga postures, breath techniques, mantras, and hand positions that must be used in a specific order.

Kundalini: The primal energy coiled at the base of the spine.

Mantra: Repetitive sounds we make to bring about a change in our consciousness.

Mudra: Yogic hand positions that stimulate centers in the brain.

Prana: Life-sustaining energy.

Pranayama: Yogic techniques of manipulating the breath.

Sadhana: A daily personal spiritual practice, usually done in the early morning hours.

Shakti: Feminine aspect of God.

Sikh: Literally "a seeker of truth," one who follows the Sikh religion, which originated in India.

Vegan: A vegetarian diet that is totally free of any animal sources, based completely on plant-based foods.

Wahe Guru: A mantra of expressing the indescribable majesty of God.

Yatra: Spiritual pilgrimage.

Yoga: Union of the individual with the Universal consciousness.

Yogi: A person who practices yoga; a master of herself.

Yogini: Feminine form of the word yogi.

INSPIRED
RESOURCES

If you would like to contact us or order any of the materials listed below, or even visit us the next time you are in the Los Angeles area, we are located at:

Golden Bridge
5901 West 3rd Street
Los Angeles, CA 90036
323-936-4172
doyoga@pacbell.net
www.GoldenBridgeYoga.com

My personal Web site is *www.Gurmukh.com*.

For reliable information on childcare issues and pregnancy, I highly suggest subscribing to *Mothering Magazine* by calling 800-984-8116 or on-line at *www.mothering.com*.

Interested in midwifery and resources for home birth? Look at the information provided by Midwife Shelley Girard at *www.socal.org*.

For more information on Michel Odent, M.D., and the Primal Research Project, contact *www.birthworks.org.*

The following videos are incredibly inspiring and educational. I recommend you watch them with your partner:

> *Birth Day*, Naoli Vinaver Lopez and family, *www.homebirthvideos.com.*
> *Birth Into Being: The Russian Waterbirth Experience*, Global Maternal/Child Health Association and Waterbirth International, P.O. Box 1400, Wilsonville, OR 97070, 800-641-BABY; *www.waterbirth.org.*
> *Giving Birth: Challenges and Choices*, Suzanne Arms, Birthing the Future, P.O. Box 830, Durango, CO 81302, 970-884-4090; *www.BirththeFuture.com.*

For expert knowledge on Chinese medicine as mentioned in the chapter "Nourish Yourself," contact Ron Teegarden at *www.dragonherbs.com.*

These books are treasures of information:

> *Spiritual Midwifery*, Ina May Gaskin, The Book Publishing Company, Summertown, TN.
> *Dear Parent: Caring for Infants with Respect*, Magda Gerber, Resources for Infant Educators, 1550 Murray Circle, Los Angeles, CA 90026, 323-663-5330. E-mail *Educarer@REI.org; www.REI.org.*

For additional information on issues surrounding circumcision, contact the National Organization of Circumcision Information Resource Centers, P.O. Box 2512, San Anselmo, CA 94979, 415-488-9883; *www.nocirc.org.*

For information on breast-feeding, call the Pump Station at 310-826-5774 in Santa Monica, CA.

This music, available through Golden Bridge, is recommended for creating a sacred space in your meditations, your birth, your life:

Sing Kaur, Vol. 1 & 2
Adi Shakti
On This Day
Sadasats
Guru Singh
I Am Thine
Humme Hum

For a copy of the song "Welcome to this World," mentioned in the chapter "A Soul Arrives," contact Jeremy Toback at *www.jeremytoback.com.*

ACKNOWLEDGMENTS

*"Teachers open the
door but you
must enter
by yourself."*

—CHINESE PROVERB

I thankfully acknowledge many in the journey of writing this book. My hope is that the book became personified as a mother calling out for all the mothers to come and stand side by side and walk this path of awareness together—tall and mighty, taking back our strength, holding our children close to us so that they might then walk free from us into the world and do something great. The word "great" will take on a new connotation as we near this new time in history; "great" will equal "from the heart."

And so from my heart, I thank so many. To Yogi Bhajan, forever, my spiritual teacher for the past thirty-two years and my guide for these ancient teachings that live in us because of him. All these years he has given and given us a way to live healthy, happy, and holy. To my beloved husband and daughter, for being my inspiration.

I am eternally grateful to Samantha Dunn, who took my handwritten notes and scattered thoughts and placed them like jewels on the page. The encouragement, guidance, and friendship of my editor, Diane Reverand, are pure gold to me. To St.

Martin's Press, which took me on in a most miraculous way. To my agent, Jane Dystel. Our due date for this manuscript fell in the week of the horrific terrorist attacks of September 2001 in New York, Washington, and Pennsylvania. She is a New Yorker all the way, and they don't come any stronger. When we all felt that the world was upside down she led the charge, saying, "Don't stop! Meet your deadline! The world needs this book more than ever."

I thank the staff and volunteers at Golden Bridge for being the cheerleaders they are, and my talented assistant, Marlene Stevens, faithful and steadfast through thick and thin, twenty-four hours a day. I thank the North Hollywood YMCA for giving me that wonderful swim each morning. That cross-crawl balanced my brain once again every day, and the kindness of the folks there fills my heart. I want to thank and bless Tej Kaur, my friend, who was always able to find the exact reference in the ancient archives to enrich this project.

I thank and bless my parents and family for making it possible to come back to this earth and for helping me to be who I am today. I bow to you all.

I appreciate the writers who have come before me and inspired, uplifted, and educated me in the birthing world. To the dedicated and tireless medical professionals who help to bring these souls onto this earth, remembering always the doctors and midwives who have put their reputations, financial security, and sometimes even their lives on the line to bring justice and freedom to mothers and children. I am so very thankful to Cindy Crawford. She is an angel not only for graciously supplying the foreword to this book, but for being a tremendous representative for women everywhere, committed to inspiring and uniting all of us in our strength and glory.

I honor each and every mama who has gone through the classes and brought all these little souls into the world. Their commitment to hard work and their awakening, sharing, and building community continue to spirit me forward. I am thankful to all who shared their thoughts and birth stories by phone, fax, or e-mail with myself and Samantha. I thank the mothers who spent an afternoon with me laughing and posing as we shot the book cover. I am grateful to Donna Burns, Alice Dodd, Jalila Salaam, and Richard Rusnak for posing for the illustrations contained

in this book. Thanks to Dawn and Clive Baillie of BLT & Associates, artists and students of Kundalini Yoga. I am forever grateful for your beautiful work on the cover.

Finally, I bow to all mothers with children, born and unborn. You hold the world in your arms and in your bellies. May the Creator forever guide and protect you and may we collectively usher in this new age of clarity and understanding.

Thank you all, and may the longtime sun shine forever and ever upon you, and may the creative force of the universe forever guide, guard, and protect you.

SAT NAM,

GURMUKH

LOS ANGELES 2001